OPTIMAL PREVENTION

BY
EDWARD R. ROSICK
DO, MPH, DABHM

Table of Contents

Optimal Prevention

How a preventive medicine approach can help you live a longer, healthier and happier life, AND avoid the five most common killer diseases.

Edward R. Rosick, DO, MPH, DABHM

DISCLAIMER

The information contained in this publication is not meant to be used, nor should it be used, to diagnose or treat any health-related or medical condition, and is in no way a substitute for the advice of a qualified healthcare provider. For diagnosis or treatment of any health or medical problem, consult your own physician. The use of any prescription medication or over-the-counter (OTC) nutritional supplement should only be done under the care and supervision of a qualified healthcare professional. The author and publisher are not responsible for any specific health or allergy needs that may require medical supervision and are not liable for any damages and/or negative consequences resulting from any treatment, action, application or preparation, to any person reading or following the information presented in this book. References are provided for informational purposes only and do not constitute endorsement of any websites or other sources. Readers should be aware that the websites listed in this book may change at any time.

About the Author

Edward R. Rosick, DO, MPH, DABIHM, is a physician and writer living in the greater Lansing MI area. Dr. Rosick is board-certified in preventive medicine, holistic medicine, and public health, and hold Master's degrees in biological sciences and public health. He has been blessed to having traveled around the world giving lectures on numerous medical and health-related topics including nutritional supplements, bioidentical hormonal replacement therapy, depression, herbal medicine and chronic stress. He has had a number of appearances on both television and radio talk shows both local and national, and is known as an informative and entertaining speaker. More information can be read at Dr. Rosick's website and blog at www.drrosick.com

Acknowledgements

Everything we do in life impacts others, and what others do impacts our lives from the moment we are conceived. The impact that many people have made upon me in my medical and writing career is overwhelming, and this book could not have been written without their help, encouragement, and kind words. Giants in the holistic medical field such as Dr. John Crisler, Dr. Jacob Teitelbaum, and Dr. Jonathan Wright have bravely fought for ideas that many in the mainstream medical world think of as heretical; yet as the years pass, they are proven correct time and time again, and I am indebted to their vision and work. I would be remiss if I did not acknowledge the help of Ms. Stephanie Six, whose hard work in manuscript preparation made this book possible. And finally, I need to thank all my patients who, over the years, have taught me far more than all the medical books and articles I have ever read on what it truly means to be a healer.

Foreword

It is truly an honor for me to offer the Foreword for my old friend, and colleague, Dr. Edward Rosick's latest addition to his impressive list of published works. Physician, musician, world traveler, writer, father, teacher, friend, collector, martial artist, medical school Departmental Chair...Dr. Rosick is truly a Man for All Seasons. He and I have enjoyed mulling over many a case over the years, and it has always impressed me how he is innately able to get right to the bottom line, the essence if you will, of the natural forces which govern how life is best maintained. Dr. Rosick has transcended the practice of medicine from being a very knowledgeable physician, and evolved into a true *healer*.

The real focus of this book is the elimination of that which is foundational to all which kills us (outside of trauma): **Inflammation**. Inflammation is the enemy within we battle on a daily basis, caused by such things as today's average diet—including, sadly, things all too commonly recommended to us by the Powers That Be—stress, lack of sleep, alcohol and other drugs, constant assault by pollutants and endocrine disrupters, even the prescription medications pushed on us by a pharmaceutical industry seemly more intent on profit than creating health. They all combine to produce "The Five Deadlies" of chronic disease: heart disease, cancer, diabetes, cerebrovascular disease, and Alzheimer's. You will know much more about all of them—and how to beat them at their own game—by the time you get to the last page of this book.

Within the covers of this book you will find, in layman's terms, abundantly referenced with true (and *applicable*) "evidence-based medicine", the simple, down to earth secrets to increasing the number of years one may enjoy the fruits of a well lived life. The rigors of the scientific method (Dr. Rosick also holds a Master of Public Health degree) mean we can't claim to prove an increase in lifespan, but we know we sure can, by own choices, lengthen *healthspan*.

Once implemented, you will find you will begin to feel better within just a few days. Inflammation can go, trending down, just that fast. Insulin levels will drop (a great marker for our state of health), and you will already know you are on the path toward improved health and happiness. These truly are changes you can make NOW...as in your very next decision(s). When Dr. Rosick says NOW, he means right NOW. Make it a habit. Make for a healthy life...for you, and for your family.

More specifically, included in this easy to read book: How to have a diet (instead of going on a diet); a beneficial list of good prescription medications; how to make more fruitful, and less wasteful, trips to the health food store; what certain lab tests mean (and don't mean); how to best talk to your doctor about your health issues and concerns, to allow the astute reader to engage in informed conversation and decision making; and more. This book is truly one stop shopping for those genuinely interested in taking away that which is bad for us, and substituting that which is good. But first things first; you need specific instructions. You need to know where to start. Were I not already a doctor, yet tasked with developing a health plan for me and my family, *Optimal Prevention* would be the next book I would read.

"Optimal Prevention" is not just a catchy phrase. It's a plan, a "recipe" if you will, a scientifically valid list of easy to follow instructions meant to empower you to keep yourself out of the doctor's office. Where conventional medicine's prescription-based therapies have proven unfruitful in curing chronic illness, Dr. Rosick's approach will stave off the chronic diseases which dampen our lives, empty our bank accounts, and just plain hurt.

In plain, easy to read terms, any medical terminology is joyfully explained, with abundant application of humor—as laughter is another good medicine—but poignant enough to stick in your mind. You will find reading this book more joy than chore. And the results are absolutely guaranteed: you CAN reduce the risk factors for chronic disease.

Dr. Rosick is a very good doctor; one who produces great results in his patients. People come to him from across the country, and all walks of life. Now we can learn, for the mere price of a book (less than an office visit), what we would otherwise only get in pieces, and after sitting in his Waiting Room, many times.

They don't teach this stuff in medical school.

—John Crisler, DO

Author "Testosterone Replacement Therapy: *A Recipe for Success*"

Introduction

Preventive Medicine: The Answer to the Health Care Crisis in twenty-first-century America.

Imagine the following scenario: a rich country of 320 million people suddenly finds its health-care budget spinning out of control. Even though 4 **trillion** dollars a year are spent on this health-care system, there are still tens of millions of people left out of it with millions more hanging on the edges. Meanwhile, deadly and debilitating chronic diseases such as cancer, Alzheimer's disease, diabetes, strokes, and heart disease affect over 100 million citizens in said country and cost hundreds of billions of dollars without counting the secondary health problems these conditions cause.

Does this country sound familiar? It should—it's the United States of America.

Now imagine a way of medical thinking that could save billions of dollars in costs. Imagine a way of practicing medicine that would save millions of people from suffering the horrors of cancer, the debilitating effects of strokes, or watching their loved ones slowly succumb to Alzheimer's.

Does this sound like a dream cooked up by politicians looking to get re-elected? Well, guess what—it isn't. In fact, it's a branch of medicine that has been neglected—and continues to be neglected—a branch called Preventive Medicine.

Preventive Medicine—one of the board-specialties that I'm certified in—is a discipline of medicine that looks at chronic diseases such as cancer, diabetes and Alzheimer's in a distinctly different way than most other medical specialties. Physicians, like myself, who are trained and board certified in preventive medicine first and foremost seek to prevent disease rather than treat symptoms of a disease once it's taken hold. For example, whereas a cardiologist tries to treat the symptoms of chest pain and shortness of breath caused by heart disease, preventive medicine specialist will try to help a person make changes to stop heart disease from occurring in the first place. We, in preventive medicine, term this 'primary prevention'—that is, helping patients do things to avoid the disease from ensuing in the first place. If the disease has already started, a preventive medicine specialist can educate a person to take measures so that the disease doesn't progress and cause debilitating symptoms (we call this 'secondary prevention'). Preventive medicine is the perfect answer to chronic diseases such as Alzheimer's, diabetes, and cancer, all of which are now the major cause of suffering and death among the rapidly increasing middle-aged and elderly population.

Chronic diseases are increasing at an alarming rate in this country despite the 4 trillion dollars a year we spend on 'health care.' Recent Gallup polls have shown that the vast majority of the public are very interested in the preventive measures they can take to protect themselves from chronic diseases such as cancer, yet are confused about what preventive measures are available and how to access them.

Go into the health section of your local bookstore—the shelves are packed with books on supplements, diets, and other things that can supposedly help you avoid chronic diseases. Unfortunately, many of these books have little scientific basis for their claims, and none were written by a doctor board certified in both preventive and holistic medicine. All except the book you are now reading.

If preventive medicine is so great, why don't all doctors do it?

You might be asking yourself, "If preventive medicine can not only save me, save the country money and help us prevent terrible diseases such as cancer and Alzheimer's, why aren't all doctors doing it?" It's a great question, and one that I've asked over the years. The sad answer is that despite all that we know about preventive medicine, despite all the lip service paid to preventive medicine by politicians, the fact is that the government does not fund **any** preventive medicine training. That's right: while all other residency training programs—the time in which young doctors train to become family physicians, cardiologists, oncologists, etc. are given federal funds (your tax dollars) to accomplish this—preventive medicine residencies have to scramble to find money from other sources since the government, in all its infinite wisdom, has decided not to fund them. "That's crazy!" some of you may be thinking—or shouting—and believe me, I've done both. But in our topsy-turvy world of twenty-first-century medicine, that's the way it is.

So, to answer the question as to why most doctors don't practice preventive medicine, the answer is sad- but simple—they're just not trained to do it. In addition, the method that we preventive medicine docs use to help our patients avoid the most common killers of Americans today consists of a lot of education and counseling. In short, we spend a significant amount of time talking to our patients.

"But that's a good thing," I can hear many of you say. "I hate it when my doctor just sits there for thirty seconds and then writes a prescription and walks out the door without hardly saying a word." Believe me, I know how you feel, and that's one reason there's such dissatisfaction with modern medicine. However, another sad fact is that reimbursement rates—in essence, what us doctors get paid—for spending time talking to patients is pennies on the dollar when compared to, say, what a surgeon gets for a one-hour long operation.

Now don't get me wrong; I have no problem with a skilled cardiologist or gifted surgeon making good money for their work—they should. What I do have a problem with is that doctors who spend time talking with their patients get the short end of the reimbursement stick. This forces most doctors in primary care fields (including preventive medicine) to abandon spending quality time with patients—in order to see more and more patients in a shorter amount of time—just so they can pay their bills.

Are DOs real doctors?

When you picked this book up, or looked at it online, you may have asked yourself "What's a D.O.?" Back in the early 1900s, there was a variety of ways you could practice medicine. However, that changed as those with the most political power—the MDs, or conventional physicians (Doctor of Medicine)—consolidated. In less than twenty years, homeopathy, naturopathy and almost all other codified medical practices were driven out of the mainstream, and only MD medical schools were allowed to flourish. However, some outlying Doctor of Osteopathy (DO) medical schools managed to stay open, and in some states, physicians with osteopathic medical degrees were still allowed to practice medicine. Today, we live in a (somewhat) more enlightened time, and both DOs and MDs are licensed to practice medicine in all fifty states.

"If you're both physicians, what's the difference?" is a question I get asked. One of the main differences is that osteopaths believe the neuromusculoskeletal structure of the human body is vital to overall health. From the first year in medical school, osteopaths learn how to correct any imbalances in this system through osteopathic manipulation. Another difference (although this difference is not nearly as much today as it was forty or fifty years ago) is that DO medical schools are—or at least were— more holistically oriented than MD medical schools. Osteopaths are taught to look at the whole person—mind, body and spirit—when considering a person's health. Because of this training and attitude, many osteopaths, including myself, realize that there are many modalities outside the realm of prescription medications and other mainstays of mainstream medicine that may help people stay healthy.

Do supplements work?

Walk through any large variety store, or even your neighborhood drug store, and you'll see aisle after aisle of vitamins, minerals, herbs and other supplements. In fact, the supplement industry in the United States generates billions of dollars every year. With over half the population of the United States stating they regularly use some type of dietary supplement, sales are only poised to increase.

"But I just read an article in some magazine that said most supplements are worthless," you might be saying. In fact, yesterday, as I was checking out at my local grocery store, I picked up a copy of *Reader's Digest* and read an article warning people about the dangers of supplements. I don't know where *Reader's Digest* gets the authors to write these articles, but I do know from writing over three hundred articles on supplements and integrative medicine that not only is the wise use of supplements **not** harmful, it can help protect you from the diseases that affect and kill millions of people every year.

If you're not sold on the usefulness of supplements, consider the issue I began this chapter with—the rising cost of medical care in this country. Recently, the Lewin

Group, a leading analytical firm, released information showing that the use of some simple, safe supplements could save over 24 billion dollars in health care costs. The major points of the study included the following:

If the 25% of American women of childbearing age who don't take folic acid would do so, the number of neural tube defects in their children could be substantially reduced, saving 1.4 billion dollars over the span of five years.

If men and women on Medicare began regularly taking calcium and vitamin D supplements, almost 800,000 hospitalizations for hip fractures could be prevented, saving more than16 billion dollars over the span of five years.

If middle-aged and elderly people began taking omega-3 fatty acid supplements, about 375,000 hospitalizations and visits to doctors for heart disease could be prevented, saving over 3 billion dollars a year.

Now, I don't know how it sounds to you, but even in a 4 trillion-dollar health-care system, 24 billion dollars sounds like a lot of money to me!

Just what is integrative medicine?

I often get asked the question—by patients, by medical students, by just about everybody—"what is integrative medicine?" Like many things in life, there are several answers to this question. One answer is that integrative (sometimes called alternative or holistic) medicine is the use of modalities—everything from supplements to energy healing—that aren't embraced by mainstream medicine. It's wise though to remember that what's ridiculed as quackery today may be embraced by main-stream medicine tomorrow, as in the use of biofeedback therapy for pain. My own personal definition of integra-tive medicine is being open minded to the different healing methods and realizing that as technologically advanced as we are today, there's still very much to learn.

Do we really need another book on preventive and integrative medicine?

If you're just skimming through this book to see if it's worth spending your hard-earned money on, you might be asking yourself, "Aren't there hundreds of books already out there on preventive medicine, with some of them written by really famous people?"

Yes, there are a lot of books out there on integrative and alternative medicine, but *Optimal Prevention* is unique in some important ways. First, it's written by a physician (me) who is board certified in both preventive and integrative medicine—as far as I know, that's a first. Second, this book focuses on how to prevent the top five killers in America today. Finally, the claims in this book aren't just mine—they're backed up by a multitude of studies done by researchers around the world.

Lies, damn lies, and statistics

Throughout this book, I'll be discussing various studies that validate the preventive and integrative medical approaches that I take with my patients. To help you understand some of these studies, I want to take a minute or two now to discuss statistics.

"There are three kinds of lies: lies, damn lies, and statistics." Anybody remember who said that famous line? It was Mark Twain, and even though he said it a long time ago, it still holds true today. Whenever you hear someone use statistics to justify something that doesn't sound right, it's probably because it isn't right. In most political seasons, you can find airwaves and newspapers filled with candidates pontificating on everything from war to food prices while using a mass of seemingly contradictory statistics to back up their claims. In both the political world and the scientific world, statistics can be bent and twisted to back up outrageous claims. Fortunately, a wise person can use a bit of common sense, as well as a basic understanding of statistics, to see through the fog of statistical lies.

As research accumulates, it can be difficult to know what's useful and what's junk. In 1976, Gene Glass came up with a way to help sort out the "good" studies from the "bad" ones. He coined his method of integrating and summarizing scientific results 'meta-analysis.' Today, the scientific and medical communities frequently use meta-analysis to get a better statistical grip on the vast amount of information available to them in the approximately 40,000 scientific and medical journals presently being published.

You may be asking, "If a bunch of studies are junk, isn't meta-analysis just a hodgepodge of junk studies?" In a properly done meta-analysis, reviewers systematically reduce things that can lead to errors, such as chance, methodological inadequacies and systematic differences in study characteristics. By doing these things, reviewers can weed out the junk science and medicine before the analysis begins. The result is much more robust than individual studies alone can provide.

When a study just isn't a study.

As you read through this book, you'll notice that I talk about different types of studies. While I don't want to bore you, it's worth a couple lines here to define some types of studies that are commonly used in research:

- Retrospective study—a study that looks backward in times; for example, we find a group of people that have cancer and then try to figure out what possibly happened in their past to cause the cancer.

- Prospective study—a study that looks forward in time; for example, we follow a group of people over a period of time and see if, say pesticide exposure causes health problems.

Practical steps you can take now

In a perfect world, the government would wake from its bureaucratic stupor and realize that putting money into preventive medicine would both save lives and money. Unfortunately, we don't live in a perfect world—in all the talk and preaching about the latest healthcare 'reform' bill, I didn't hear anyone talk meaningfully about preventive or integrative medicine. Therefore, it's up to you to make the changes that will make preventive medicine the way we practice medicine in this country.

On a personal level, read this book from cover to cover and implement whatever is right for you. On a larger scale, learn more about prevention and then educate your friends, your relatives, and even your physician. Finally, write and call your congressional representatives and senators at both the state and national level—if there's one thing politicians respond to, it's an active and engaged populace!

Chapter 1: It's All in Your Head

Have you seen the Jim Carrey movie *Eternal Sunshine of the Spotless Mind*? Don't feel bad if you haven't—it wasn't one of Carrey's usual blockbuster slapstick comedies. In a nutshell, the movie looked at the consequences of being able to erase unpleasant memories. At times, the notion of being able to erase painful thoughts and memories that cause pain and anguish may seem like a good thing, but in reality, there would be significant drawbacks. By being able to hit 'delete' and erase your memories, you would literally get rid of part of your life, because what are our lives if not a dearly held collection of memories? To me, the disease that does this is Alzheimer's disease. It robs you of your memories and mind, and therefore ultimately robs you of you. Along with cancer, it's one of the most horrible diagnoses I can give to my patients. Unfortunately, it's one that is becoming an epidemic in the twenty-first century.

Alzheimer's disease: A killer of the soul

A German neuropathologist, Dr. Alois Alzheimer, gave the first clinical description of the disease that eventually bore his name. Alzheimer's disease, the most common cause of dementia in those aged 65 or older, is characterized by a progressive decline in cognition and memory. Current statistics indicate that this debilitating condition affects over 15 million people worldwide. With the rapidly aging population in the United States (it's estimated that 30% of the population will be 65 or older by the year 2050), at least 14 million people in the U.S. will be stricken with Alzheimer's during the coming decades. For all these people, the twenty-first century will not hold the memories of a long and happy life, but of confusion and uncertainty.

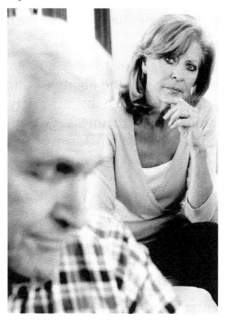

Alzheimer's causes memory loss in multiple ways

The terrible nature of Alzheimer's disease is two-fold: not only does it rob you of your memory, but it also does so in an insidious, conspiratorial way. Alzheimer's generally starts out as mild memory loss, just another sign of getting old. Who among us doesn't forget where the car keys are now and then? However, as the disease progresses, people will often start having more memory problems, so much so that they may require assistance with everyday tasks such as chores, grooming, and dressing. Finally, severe and profound dementia sets in, leading to a person with Alzheimer's being unable to communicate, reason, or remember. People in the final stages of Alzheimer's are often bedridden and require constant, round-the-clock care.

What's the difference between dementia, Alzheimer's, and mild cognitive impairment?

A question I hear from my patients goes something like this: "Another doctor told me my aunt [or mother, father, etc.] is developing dementia. Does this mean that she has Alzheimer's?"

It's a good question and one to clear up right now. For the record: Dementia (loss of the ability to think, remember, and reason) can be caused by a variety of factors—infections, trauma, or Alzheimer's. AD, Alzheimer's Dementia, is the most common form of dementia. So all Alzheimer's is dementia, but not all dementia is Alzheimer's.

Another question that's been coming up more often is: "My friend was told by her doctor that she has mild cognitive impairment [MCI] and now she's convinced she's going to get Alzheimer's. Is this true?" This one is a little trickier to answer.

MCI represents a process whereby patients show a statistically significant decline in their memory when compared to other patients of the same age and sex. In contrast to patients with Alzheimer's, people with MCI generally have no other cognitive complaints—that is, they have no problems driving, dressing themselves, cooking dinner, etc. It should be noted that the study of MCI is still new; there's no consensus among mainstream (or even integrative) physicians on what does and what does not comprise MCI.

Studies show that people with MCI do not automatically go on to develop Alzheimer's. In the Canadian Study of Health of Aging, of 296 men and women, 29% remained stable—that is, they did not further deteriorate into Alzheimer's, while 10% recovered—that is, regained normal memory and cognitive function. In a more recent study published, Italian researchers examined 52 elderly men and women (mean age of 72 years) with MCI over a 2-month to 3-year period. The researchers found that almost 54% of the patients remained stable in terms of their memory retention, while 17 percent of them regained normal brain function.

"So even if I have MCI, are you saying that I don't have to worry about Alzheimer's?" is a reasonable question many of you are probably asking. Unfortunately, that's not the case. Preliminary data indicates that about 10% or so of people with MCI will go on to develop Alzheimer's versus 2% of the general population. Because of this statistically increased risk, I believe that it's imperative that we in the medical community—both mainstream and integrative—be aggressive in formalizing tests and standards to determine if a person is developing MCI. Unfortunately, that day isn't here yet. Because subtle changes in memory and cognition happen to all of us at one point or another—and especially as we age—defining who has MCI remains a critical challenge. New screening tests—such as the Montreal Cognitive Assessment—are being developed to help health care providers have a rapid, sensitive tool to assess memory and MCI. In addition, imaging studies like magnetic resonance imaging (MRI) have shown that people with MCI, like those with Alzheimer's, tend to have a loss of cells in the hippocampus, an area of the brain that's critically important to memory formation.

Because of this small but statistical risk between MCI and Alzheimer's, the American Academy of Neurology has recommended that people be monitored closely if their physician feels that they have MCI. Since it's known that early detection and treatment of Alzheimer's is critically important, it only makes sense to think that if you are at risk for MCI, the sooner you can take steps to prevent it's progression, the better. The bottom line to me is that whether or not MCI leads to Alzheimer's, it's imperative to recognize the danger and begin a program that very well might be able to delay—or even prevent, MCI, and therefore, Alzheimer's.

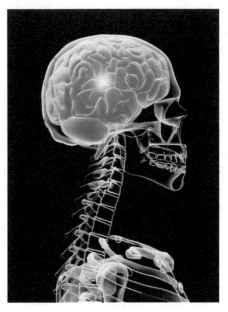

What occurs in a brain with Alzheimer's?

Like other chronic diseases discussed in this book, Alzheimer's doesn't have one single cause; rather, it's a "multi-factorial disease." The bottom line is that while we in the medical world don't really know what causes Alzheimer's, we think that there's a number of processes going on that, in the end, cause the disease or at least lead up to it.

Most medical researchers think there are at least four changes that occur in the brain in of someone with Alzheimer's. In no particular order, those four changes are as follows:

- A build-up of destructive deposits known as beta-amyloid plaque (protein) (made up of stuff called beta-amyloid) in and around the brain cells. As this beta-amyloid plaque builds up, it literally gunks up the brain. As you can imagine, this is not a good thing.

- Damage to brain cells by free radicals. Free radicals aren't the latest heavy metal band or leftover hippie rock group from the 1970s, but rather molecules formed in all of our bodies when food and oxygen gets turned into energy. While your body can, at least to a degree, neutralize the damaging effects of free radicals, a slowdown in our personal anti-free radical defense mechanisms occurs slowly as we age, leading to the damage of cells, tissues, and organs. You might be thinking to yourself "how do these free radicals cause damage?" The answer is through a chemical process known as oxidation. This idea—that oxidative damage brought about by free radicals is a major factor in age-related human diseases such as Alzheimer's—was formally proposed by Dr. Denham Harman way back in1954.

- Decrease in levels of the brain chemical acetylcholine, a chemical that is vitally important for memory formation and retention. As I'll talk about in a minute, medications that increase the levels of acetylcholine levels are the mainstay of the modern medical treatment of Alzheimer's.

- Inflammatory changes—much like the inflammation that occurs in your muscles after you exercise hard, which, like oxidative damage, can lead to brain cell death.

AGEs and aluminum: Two more crucial pieces of the Alzheimer's puzzle.

Besides those four processes described above, there are other things that we're just starting to learn about which may bring about Alzheimer's.

One of these is something you've probably never heard about—AGEs, and another that you have heard about and which surrounds us in our technological society—aluminum. Let's talk about AGEs first.

Advanced glycation end-products (AGEs) are molecules that may be just as important as free radicals in playing a key role in Alzheimer's (and other diseases that I'll talk about later in the book). AGEs are formed in your body by the interaction between carbohydrates and proteins in a process known to chemists as the Maillard reaction. This widespread, but little known reaction is what gives cooked foods their unique texture, taste, and smell. When you're enjoying the delectable aromas of a Thanksgiving turkey, remember to thank Mr. Maillard!

The reason that AGEs are such a big thing (besides their cool acronym) is because they cause a process known as protein cross-linking, which is generally a bad thing, especially when it happens inside your body. When proteins cross link, they don't work as well as they should. Since proteins are essential to life and living, AGEs can and do cause a whole lot of damage inside you, including and even causing Alzheimer's.

The deadly connection between AGEs and Alzheimer's

So why do some researchers think that AGEs may be part of the Alzheimer puzzle? For one thing, it's been shown that beta-amyloid plaques contain significant amounts of AGEs. In addition, new research has shown that while AGEs are present in higher amounts in the brains of patients who have died from Alzheimer's, they are also formed early on in the disease process. This discovery has led some researchers to think that AGE formation represents an early event in disease development.

Finally, while I hate to be the bearer of bad news, here's some that you need to know—while AGEs are destructive on their own, when combined with free radicals these two bad boys of human biochemistry wreak even more havoc in your body. Research shows that free radicals are involved in AGE formation; and then, in a vicious cycle, AGEs cause more oxidative stress. As these AGEs and free radicals build up in your body, damage and destruction increase down to the level of your DNA leading to Alzheimer's and other conditions associated with growing old.

Is your kitchen giving you Alzheimer's?

One of the toughest jobs I have as a physician of integrative and preventive medicine is separating fact from fantasy. It would be much easier to believe, like many of my mainstream medical brethren do, that if a report isn't from the *New England Journal of Medicine* (which I read every week), then it just isn't true.

However, I consider it part of my duty to help educate my patients on what medical information—mainstream or otherwise—they should take seriously. Take for example the reports that high levels of aluminum—a metal that's in everything from your frying pans to antiperspirants—may be a cause of Alzheimer's. If you ask most mainstream doctors about this you'll probably get a "those reports are nonsense!" response. However, some reputable epidemiological studies have shown that higher levels of aluminum in drinking water may be an independent risk factor for developing Alzheimer's. Over an eight-year period, researchers in France studied the possible connection between aluminum in drinking water and Alzheimer's over 3,000 men and women. The researchers concluded "high concentrations of aluminum in drinking water may be a risk factor for Alzheimer's." Because of this, and other studies, I've changed all my cookware to either stainless steel or copper and I urge you to do the same.

The link between baloney and Alzheimer's

A baloney sandwich—or better yet, a fried baloney sandwich—used to be one of my favorite foods for lunch as a kid. Unfortunately, that snack—and any other food preserved with chemicals called nitrates and nitrites—may be one of the causes for the rising rate of Alzheimer's. A study released in the *Journal of Alzheimer's Disease* looked at the disturbing link between the rising rate of Alzheimer's and the rising use of nitrates and nitrites. While nitrates and nitrites are known carcinogens, this new research regarding nitrates and Alzheimer's—in my humble opinion—should put the final nail in the coffin regarding the use of nitrates and nitrites. My advice is to be a smart shopper: if the food you're thinking of purchasing has one of these toxins in it, put it back!

Are Alzheimer's and heart disease connected?

As if it isn't bad enough to develop Alzheimer's, some researchers now think that this emerging epidemic is intimately connected with another epidemic top killer in America—heart disease.

A report in the *Proceedings of the New York Academy of Sciences* has shown that hypoxia—the reduction in the amount of oxygen to the brain—may be a trigger for Alzheimer's.

The authors of this important research study have shown that hypoxia causes higher levels of oxidative stress and increase in the activity of a gene that controls production of beta-amyloid (the stuff that gunks up the brain). In addition, hypoxic conditions also bring about higher levels of oxidative stress. In other words, hypoxia may very well set off a chain of events that leads to Alzheimer's. Because conditions like heart disease are a cause of brain hypoxia, there may in fact be a nasty connection between two of the largest killers of Americans today.

And finally... Alzheimer's may be type-3 diabetes

A little while ago I told you that Alzheimer's is a "multifactorial disease," and I wasn't kidding. In fact, there are now some scientists who are proposing that Alzheimer's is another type of diabetes. (If you don't know much about diabetes, feel free to jump to chapter four for an introduction—I won't mind!).

If this sounds like science fiction and leaves you thinking, "c'mon, Doc, how can something that raises your blood sugar and insulin levels like diabetes have anything to do with Alzheimer's?" you should know that there are some impressive lines of evidence that back this notion. One widely referenced work is the Rotterdam Study, where researchers examined 6,370 elderly men and women over an average period of 2 years. During that time, the researchers noted which subjects developed Alzheimer's and which had diabetes. They discovered that having diabetes almost doubled the risk of dementia.

Another study, published by researchers at the Mayo Clinic, also looked at the association between type-2 diabetes (and its associated high insulin levels) and the risk of Alzheimer's. Researchers followed 683 men and women and examined them for signs of Alzheimer's and increased insulin levels. As in the *Rotterdam Study*, the authors of this study found that high insulin levels, which are intimately connected with type-2 diabetes, were significantly associated with a higher risk of developing Alzheimer's.

A paper in the respected medical journal *Archives of Neurology* explained why high insulin levels may be closely linked to Alzheimer's. In this study, researchers showed that by mimicking high insulin levels (such as those seen in patients with insulin resistance and type-2 diabetes) in 16 healthy men ranging in age from 55 to 81, there was elevation of inflammatory markers and beta-amyloid in the brain.

Can an upset stomach lead to Alzheimer's?

There's probably not many of you who haven't occasionally experienced an upset stomach and/or heartburn that caused you to take a medicine like Tagamet or Zantac. Known as H2 blockers, these medications, which reduce stomach acid, are available both as prescriptions and over-the-counter. Unfortunately, recent data published in the *Journal of the American Geriatrics* shows that these commonly used medications may contribute to mental decline in the elderly.

In this study on aging, researchers at Indiana University examined the connection between H2 blockers and cognitive impairment in 1,558 elderly (aged 65 and older) African Americans. What they found was alarming: among long-term users of H2 medications there was a 2.4 times higher chance of developing some form of mental decline. While these results need to be confirmed, it again emphasizes what I tell my patients—if there's no good reason to be taking medications for a long period of time, then don't do it!

Is there any good news regarding Alzheimer's?

By now, you might be thinking, "c'mon, Dr. Rosick, there has to be some good news about Alzheimer's—isn't the government spending millions of dollars to find a cure?"

Of course the government (using all of our hard-earned tax dollars) and multinational pharmaceutical companies are spending tens, if not hundreds of millions of dollars to find a treatment for Alzheimer's disease, but the news here isn't very good: Prescription drugs for Alzheimer's are limited in their effectiveness. The most common Alzheimer's drug is called acetylcholinesterase inhibitors. What they do is increase the amount of acetylcholine in the brain, which then leads to better memory retention. Although these drugs lead to a modest decrease in the rate of progression of Alzheimer's, they do not stop the disease. Another Alzheimer's medication, memantine, works on the part of the brain called NMDA receptors, but like the acetylcholinesterase inhibitors, it doesn't stop the progression of the disease.

Prescription medications for Alzheimer's

Generic Name **Brand Name**

Donepezil Aricept

Rivastigmine Exelon

Galantamine Razadyne

Memantine Namenda

Why isn't more money put into the prevention of Alzheimer's?

For years I've asked why more money isn't being put into preventing Alzheimer's, and I haven't gotten a good answer. To me, Alzheimer's should be one of the top five diseases we should focus on preventing. As I just said, the prescription medications we have for Alzheimer's aren't that good; in fact, they generally only slow the disease for 6-12 months. Second, it has been shown that by the time Alzheimer's—even in mild form— is diagnosed, there's already been a 30% to 50% loss of brain cells.

But alas, like in other chronic diseases I'll talk about in this book, modern mainstream medicine seems hell-bent on finding a cure for Alzheimer's, which is fine and good, except for the fact that finding the cure is proving quite elusive. Meanwhile, millions of people and their families are suffering while effective preventive measures are staring us right in the face. So, if the government won't try to point you in the right direction toward preventing this devastating disease, then I will.

'Use it or lose it' applies to many body parts, including your brain

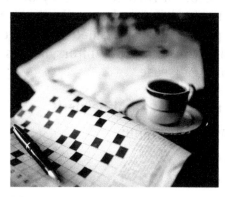

You've probably heard the saying "use it or lose it." And, like many other hokey-sounding old sayings, this one has got a lot of truth to it. If you don't exercise, your muscles will waste away, causing a condition called sarcopenia. If you don't practice skills you learned as a child, all those piano lessons your parents forced you to take will go to waste. If you don't have sex, your... anyway, you get the idea.

The same is true with your brain. If you don't use it—if you don't keep yourself mentally engaged in something as you grow older, then you're at higher risk for developing Alzheimer's. I can't tell you why this is so, but there are enough studies out there, even in such mainstream medical journals such as the *Journal of the American Medical Association,* to make me a firm believer in mental exercise.

What do I mean by mental exercise? I mean things like reading, writing poetry, doing crossword puzzles, playing cards, or anything else that requires some form of thinking.

While we're on the subject of exercise, it's not just mental exercise that can help prevent Alzheimer's: physical exercise has also been shown to do so. Just as with mental exercise, we in the medical community are at a loss to explain just how this works, but it does. Am I saying you need to go out and pump iron seven days a week? Not at all. Most studies on exercise and Alzheimer's show that just light exercising (such as walking, riding a stationary bike or, lifting light weights), 3 three times a week can make a significant difference in preventing Alzheimer's. Exercise is one of the most important things that you can do to ward off Alzheimer' and other members of the big deadly five.

Stop your headache, stop Alzheimer's?

A few short years ago, the medical community was excited about the possibility that aspirin and other NSAIDs (yes, another annoying acronym; this one stands for non-steroidal anti-inflammatory drugs) such as naproxen and ibuprofen may be useful in both preventing and treating Alzheimer's. A review paper in 2005 looked at the results of multiple studies using NSAIDs to prevent Alzheimer's and came to the conclusion that these commonly used drugs do have the potential to protect against Alzheimer's.

So, does this mean you should start gulping NSAIDS like candy every day? Well, maybe not. A study published in the journal *Archives of Neurology* on over 6,000 women showed that those who had a family history of Alzheimer's and who took low-dose aspirin, naproxen, or celecoxib (the prescription anti-inflammatory) were not protected against the development of Alzheimer's.

"Now wait a minute, Dr. Rosick," you might be thinking. "Just a second ago you said that a bunch of studies showed that NSAIDs protect against Alzheimer's, and now you're saying they don't?"

No. What I'm saying is that this is a perfect example of science being imperfect. My interpretation of the research is that yes, certain NSAIDs, especially ibuprofen, may help prevent Alzheimer's, either by reducing inflammation in the brain or stopping the formation of beta-amyloid plaques, or something else we have yet to fathom. However, other NSAIDs, like celecoxib and naproxen, may not provide any protection, even though they may work well at targeting your headache.

Natural approaches to preventing Alzheimer's

Ginkgo biloba: an ancient tree for a modern day epidemic

If there's any supplement that ranks number one in the fight against Alzheimer's, then that title should go to Ginkgo biloba. Gingko has been used for at least the past 5,000 years for a variety of medical conditions, including age-related memory loss. Modern science is finally catching up with the wisdom of our elders by showing that ginkgo extracts can provide remarkable protection against the four most common pathological changes seen in the brains of patients with Alzheimer's.

In terms of maintaining optimal acetylcholine levels, a recent study reported that ginkgo protects the brain against age-related losses of the brain cells that produce acetylcholine. The same study reported that ginkgo increases the amount of acetylcholine in the hippocampus (and no, this has nothing to do with hippopotami!), a part of your brain that is vitally important to memory.

Other studies have shown that in addition to keeping your acetylcholine levels high, ginkgo extracts can protect brain cells in the hippocampus against beta-amyloid, (those proteins that causes plaque to form in the brain). This is in contrast to prescription medications for Alzheimer's disease, which do nothing to prevent beta-amyloid-induced damage.

Ginkgo is also a potent antioxidant (remember those dastardly free radicals?). A study in the journal *Phytochemical Research* reported that standardized gingko extract increases the levels of antioxidant enzymes. Finally, with its ability to act as an anti-inflammatory agent, researchers are now postulating that another way ginkgo combats Alzheimer's may be mediated by its anti-inflammatory action.

With this potent list of its many anti-Alzheimer's activities, it should come as no surprise that ginkgo is now used by many physicians (me included) to treat Alzheimer's patients. However, since this book is about prevention, we'll focus on that, and there the news is also good. Well, 'good' in the sense that our kind and benevolent government is actually doing a study on ginkgo's use in the prevention of Alzheimer's. Unfortunately, the news is that like most government endeavors, this one is going to take forever—or at least a few more years— before it gives us any answers.

I'm all for the government finally using our money on studies such as this. However, I'm not willing to wait—and I'm certainly not willing to have my patients' wait—for a study that's going to take such a long time to complete. With all the available evidence out there right now, it's prudent to start using ginkgo as a preventive measure against Alzheimer's, especially if you have a family history of this dreaded disease.

Death to free radicals!

As you read this book, you're going to find I spend a good deal of time talking about free radicals and antioxidants, and for good reason: Besides being implicated in the

Alzheimer's disease, free radicals are also culprits in cancer, heart disease, diabetes... you get the picture.

I know some of my mainstream medical colleagues are going to say, "Aren't antioxidant supplements just modern-day snake oil?" My answer is no, especially when it comes to your brain. The simple fact is that while your brain generates a whole lot of free radicals, it's not very well equipped to handle this excess load. In people who are at high risk for Alzheimer's (those over the age of 65 or who have with a family history of the disease), it seems clear that taking antioxidant supplements is a very reasonable way to help prevent Alzheimer's.

Now, don't just take my word for it—look at the studies like the one done in Switzerland. In this work, researchers looked at 442 elderly patients and found a direct correlation between the blood levels of two common antioxidants (beta-carotene and alpha-tocopherol) and memory retention. Another study published in the widely respected journal *Archives of Neurology*, reported on the risk of Alzheimer's in people who took antioxidant supplements. Researchers in this study examined over four thousand elderly people (65 or older) and found that those who used supplemental vitamin C and vitamin E (two well-known antioxidants) had a reduced risk of Alzheimer's. It doesn't get much clearer than that!

Resveratrol: a gift from the grape

Besides 'traditional' antioxidants such as vitamins C and E, other natural antioxidant supplements that have significant antioxidant properties are showing their worth in the fight against Alzheimer's. One of the most exciting of these supplements is resveratrol. This compound is a naturally derived substance found in the skin and seeds of grapes. There is significant amounts of resveratrol in red wine; however, it is not found to any appreciable degree in white wine, (sorry to all you white wine lovers), since white wine is made from the juice of the grapes, not the skin.

While research on resveratrol isn't as advanced as with the research on other supplements, I still think resveratrol should be included in our anti-Alzheimer's list. Multiples lab studies have shown resveratrol to be a potent antioxidant in its own right. In addition, recent studies have shown that resveratrol can protect brain cells against beta-amyloid and free radical toxicity. While I'm certainly looking forward to human studies on resveratrol, I still think it's worthwhile to take as a resveratrol supplement—or, as I like to do, have a glass of nice red wine at dinner—to help ward off Alzheimer's.

Vitamin D—the sunshine vitamin that keeps your brain illuminated and Alzheimer's free.

When my patients ask me what vitamin is one that they absolutely must take, my answer is automatic: vitamin D. It seems that every month another study is published showing that low vitamin D levels are implicated in all chronic diseases such as Alzheimer's and cancer, and yet our government still hasn't raised its woefully inadequate recommended daily allowance (RDA).

An article in the *Journal of Geriatric Psychiatry and Neurology* examined the serum concentration of vitamin D and cognitive impairment among 1,766 men and women aged 65 or older in England. The researchers showed that—after excluding other risk factors for Alzheimer's—having a low level of vitamin D in your bloodstream puts you at a significantly increased risk for developing dementia. Because of this and other studies, I routinely check the levels of vitamin D in all my patients—young and old alike—and have found that a vast majority of them are vitamin-D deficient - or at least until I have them taking a vitamin D supplement!

Drink pomegranate juice for a healthy mind.

One of the hottest natural drinks on the market right now is pomegranate juice, and this time, the hype might live up to its potential. Pomegranate juice is high in chemicals called polyphenols, which just happen to be potent antioxidants (resveratrol is also a polyphenol). Because of this, scientists are already looking at how this staple on many people's breakfast menu may help prevent certain diseases like Alzheimer's. In early studies on mice, researchers showed that mice given pomegranate juice had significantly less accumulation of beta-amyloid in their hippocampus. While it's always wise to remember that what happens in lab animals might not work in humans, I certainly think it can't hurt to have a glass of pomegranate juice every day.

Glutathione—a triad of important amino acids for your brain keeps your antioxidants recharged.

Glutathione, made of the three amino acids glutamine, glycine, and cysteine, has been shown for the past 90 years to be one of the most widespread and important substances in the human body. Glutathione has multiple functions, including detoxification of noxious substances such as heavy metals and pesticides; regulation of immune response; maintenance of sperm maturation; regulation of the inflammatory response; and last—but certainly not least—maintenance of the body's antioxidant defense system. Glutathione's antioxidant properties are what we integrative-medicine docs like myself are so keen on—that and studies showing that patients who have higher blood levels of glutathione show lower rates of Alzheimer's.

Because of studies like these—as well as glutathione's known antioxidant properties—I wholeheartedly promote keeping your glutathione levels at optimal levels.

However, remember to not waste your money on taking glutathione supplements. Even though some less-than-ethical supplement makers will tell you otherwise, your body can't absorb glutathione, because we humans possess an enzyme (Gamma-glutamyl-transferase) that breaks down glutathione in the gut. Studies have shown that even at oral doses of 3,000 grams, glutathione supplements don't raise your blood levels of glutathione. However, don't despair—there are multiple ways to effectively increase your glutathione levels through a variety of other safe and natural supplements including:

Whey protein: a former by-product can boost your glutathione levels

During the process of making cheese, by-products are formed that once were considered waste products. One of those "waste" products—whey—is now known to be an extremely important functional food that can confer a number of health benefits. Whey is thought to produce this activity by providing a rich source of the sulfur-containing amino acids cysteine and methionine, which can lead to increased glutathione levels; in fact, studies have shown that taken orally, whey supplements can substantially increase plasma glutathione levels.

Acetyl-L-carnitine and alpha lipoic acid

These two vital antioxidants for maintaining brain function and optimal glutathione levels are remarkably safe supplements that should get more press in regards to their potential of preventing Alzheimer's. Alpha-lipoic acid, found in small amounts in some foods (such as spinach, potatoes, and red meat), is a remarkable antioxidant that is able to regenerate other antioxidants, including vitamin E and glutathione.

Acetyl-L-carnitine (ALC) is vital to the energy production in each and every cell in your brain and body. Acetyl-L-carnitine is also an antioxidant, a potent inhibitor of AGEs, and a rejuvenator of glutathione. Because of these varied actions, acetyl-L-carnitine has been used to treat problems ranging from infertility to Alzheimer's.

Due to the fantastic safety profiles of these two, alpha-lipoic acid and acetyl-L-carnitine are on my top of my recommended list when it comes to supplements used to fight Alzheimer's.

Folic acid isn't just for a baby's brain anymore!

I hope that by the now the word is out to pregnant women everywhere about folic acid. This important B-vitamin is absolutely essential for the optimal development of a fetus's brain; if you're pregnant, or trying to get pregnant, please be sure to get at least 800 micrograms (not milligrams) of folic acid every single day.

"But I'm not pregnant," you might be saying. "In fact, I'm a gray-haired 65-year-old man. Why are you talking about pregnant women and babies?" Good point, and here's the answer: studies have shown that among 49,000 elderly women and men (70-79 years old or older), those who had the highest levels of folic acid intake had the lowest risk of developing cognitive decline as seen in those with Alzheimer's. Because of these and other studies, I recommend to almost all my elderly patients to take a good B-complex vitamin that contains at least 800 micrograms of folic acid.

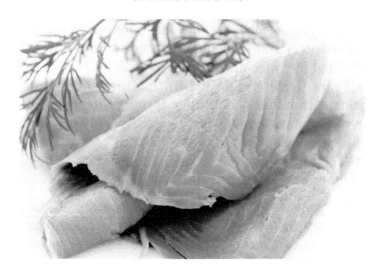

Omega-3 fatty acids from fish oil are vitally important for both heart and brain health

Some of my patients who come to see me are at first skeptical about the benefits of using supplements. A common statement is "I don't want to take a lot of supplements, so tell me which ones are the most important and I'll start with those." For those people—and, actually, to just about everyone else I see—I emphasize the importance of omega-3 fatty acids.

Omega-3 fatty acids are not fats, but are precursors to fats in our bodies. Fish oil contains two very special omega-3 fatty acids: Eicosapentaenoic acid (EPA) and docosahexaenoic acid (DHA). EPA and DHA are known as essential fatty acids, because the human body cannot produce them, yet they are required for many necessary bodily functions, including lipid metabolism, blood pressure regulation, immune modulation, and brain development. Without consumption of food or supplements containing omega-3 fatty acids, optimal health is simply not possible.

In my opinion, there is now indisputable evidence that supplementation with omega-3 fatty acids can prevent and treat a variety of chronic diseases, including heart disease (you'll learn a whole lot more about this in the next chapter) and Alzheimer's. In one study, researchers examined 899 men and women over an average period of 9.1 years to determine if DHA had a protective action against Alzheimer's and other forms of dementia. What the researchers found was that those people who had the highest levels of DHA in their bloodstream had an amazing 47% reduction in their risk of developing Alzheimer's and other forms of dementia.

Other studies add to the impressive résumé of omega-3 fatty acids. In one study looking at over 2,000 men and women, researchers showed that those people who had a higher intake of omega-3s had a substantially reduced risk of cognitive decline as seen in those with Alzheimer's.

Another study examined 210 men (with ages between 70 and 89) and showed that those who ate more fish high in omega-3s showed significantly less decline in their cognitive abilities when compared to men who had low intakes of omega-3 fatty acids.

Some of you might be asking the question "do you know exactly how fish oil protects against Alzheimer's?" The answer is "not exactly." We do know that one possible way omega-3 fatty acids from fish oil may accomplish this is through their action on beta-amyloid formation in the brain. Some groundbreaking studies have shown that in mice, increased consumption of DHA-enhanced feed decreased brain beta-amyloid levels by 70%. These results suggest that fish oil may protect against Alzheimer's by limiting beta-amyloid production, accumulation, and toxicity. Who could be against that?

Having optimal hormone levels is crucial in the prevention of chronic diseases including Alzheimer's.

You want to get your mainstream medical doctor all cranked up? Just mention that you're interested in using bio-identical hormones to maintain your health. Chances are the she or he will tell you that not only are bio-identical hormones worthless, they also cause all sorts of nasty problems like heart disease and cancer. Unfortunately, they're dead wrong. In fact, exciting new data is coming to light showing that maintaining optimal hormonal levels is crucial in the fight against chronic diseases like Alzheimer's.

A great review article published in the journal *Frontiers of Neuroendocrinology*, reported on the close association between optimal levels of estrogen in women and testosterone in men and the reduced risk of developing Alzheimer's. I'm not going to go into detail —feel free to download the article to read for yourself—but the bottom line is that low levels of these crucial hormones very likely puts you at risk for developing Alzheimer's (and other chronic diseases that I'll discuss in later chapters). Because of these and other studies, I routinely offer hormone testing to all my patients and if they're at a low level, I discuss with them supplementing with bio-identical (not synthetic, which are deadly) hormones.

The list continues to grow...

Besides fish oil, resveratrol, antioxidants, and the other natural supplements I've talked about, here are a few more things that very well may help us all avoid Alzheimer's. While the research behind these substances might not be as robust as the research behind those I've already listed, I think these substances are safe enough — and have enough potential to prevent Alzheimer's—to be included here.

Coffee

That's right, America's favorite morning drink may not just be a way to keep our brains alert longer than we thought—it may keep us from getting Alzheimer's. A study of 54 men and women (aged 50 and up), showed those who had a higher caffeine intake from coffee had a statistically significant decreased risk of developing Alzheimer's. For me, research like this makes my morning espresso taste even better!

Curcumin

Are any of you out there fans of East Asian food? If so, you might be protecting yourself against Alzheimer's via the curry spice turmeric called curcumin: a rich source of polyphenols. In fact, as you'll see in a later chapter, this spice may be important in protecting you from other deadly diseases such as cancer. But since this chapter is on Alzheimer's, let's focus our attention there. So far, studies on curcumin have so far been limited to the lab and animal tests, but the results have been nothing short of impressive. Curcumin has been shown to not only be a potent polyphenol (remember those?) antioxidant, but also has significant anti-inflammatory properties. In mice, curcumin has been shown to be able to reduce levels of beta-amyloid. With this impressive résumé, feel quite free to use this tasty spice each and every day.

Green tea

It seems you can't go a week without hearing some more good news about green tea. While I always caution my patients to not believe everything they hear and read (as well as see on TV), the science behind the hype regarding green tea is very impressive. Green tea is loaded with a polyphenol antioxidant called epigallocatechin-3-gallate (don't worry, I don't expect you to memorize this!) that's been shown in multiple lab and animal studies to significantly decrease oxidative stress on the brain and to inhibit formation of beta-amyloid plaques. A review article on the benefits of green tea highlights the ways in which this drink, consumed by millions across the globe, provides protection against Alzheimer's. Another study showed that green tea contains chemicals that can ward off the nasty effects of beta-amyloid in your brain. If you're not a coffee drinker (or even if you are), think about having a cup or two of green tea every day so that when you're 80 or 90 years old you'll still be able to think.

Strawberries and spinach

I know that some of you may already be thinking, "Come on, Dr. Rosick, what do strawberries and spinach have to do with each other?" A good question deserving of a good answer, and the answer is flavonoids, a potent antioxidants that are a type of polyphenol. (Are you getting the feeling that polyphenols might be important in keeping us healthy? Me too!). Like curcumin and green tea, studies on the protective action of flavonoids against Alzheimer's have been confined to the lab and to animal studies, but that shouldn't deter you from eating strawberries, spinach and colorful fruits and vegetables like strawberries and spinach. Who knows, maybe Popeye was more right then we knew!

A handful of walnuts a day may help keep Alzheimer's away

Enjoy foods like walnuts, almonds, and cashews? I certainly do, and now research is showing us that nuts—at least walnuts—can help protect your brain against Alzheimer's and cognitive decline. A recent article in the *Journal of Nutrition and Aging* examined data from the National Health and Nutrition Examination Survey (NHANES) and found that those adults—young, old, and in-between—who ate a couple handfuls of walnuts a day showed higher testing in cognitive testing including symbol digit substitution, single digit learning, and story recall.

Zeaxanthin: good for your eyes, good for your brain

Have you heard that carrots are good for your eyes? Like so many other common stories that mainstream medicine has frowned upon, this story is very much rooted in fact: carrots are high in carotenoids, bio-nutrients that have been shown in multiple studies to contribute to optimal eye health as well as being able to prevent some devastating eye diseases such as macular degeneration. Now, research has shown that one of these carotenoids, zeaxanthin (pronounced zee-uh-zan-thin), may be important in maintaining a healthy brain and avoiding Alzheimer's. Researchers in France conducted a nine-year study on over 1,300 elderly men and women. The results of their study showed that those men and women who had a decline in their cognitive abilities, which is often an early sign of Alzheimer's, also had the lowest levels of zeaxanthin in their blood. While more studies need to be done, it's certainly a wise idea to up your intake of carrots and other foods that are high in carotenoids to protect both your eyes and your brain.

Carnosine

Last, but certainly not least, is carnosine, an extremely safe compound that's composed of the amino acids beta-alanine and L-histidine and should be on your list when it comes to supplements to prevent Alzheimer's. Carnosine may help prevent Alzheimer's by inhibiting AGE formation and fighting free radicals. It has also been shown (at least in lab studies) to protect against the ravages of beta-amyloid formation. While more definitive human studies need to be done to confirm its potential, I see no reason why carnosine, given its safe nature, shouldn't be used in the fight to prevent Alzheimer's.

The time to prevent Alzheimer's is now!

As a teenager, I watched my grandfather, a man who had immigrated to America after being wounded in Europe during World War I, who had worked the iron ore mines of Minnesota, and had eventually retired on a small farm in Taylor, Michigan—in short, a man who had worked hard to find the 'American Dream'—slowly and horribly die from Alzheimer's disease. As a physician, I re-live those days with each and every patient I see with this horrible disease. However, with a concerted effort from our public health programs, there's no reason that the number of people who develop Alzheimer's can't be significantly reduced. Yet until the day comes when the government puts as much effort and money into preventing deadly diseases such as Alzheimer's as it puts into things like wars and wasteful spending, I think we should all take the initiative to protect our minds from the ravages of time. It's the wise person who carefully considers and talks to their doctors about all of the options—behavioral, dietary, and supplements— I've listed below in this and following chapters in order to prevent the twenty-first centuries burgeoning epidemics.

Strategies to prevent Alzheimer's

<u>**1-Behavioral Tips**</u>

- Exercise your mind. Do cross word puzzles, play cards, read books, and avoid television as much as possible!

- Exercise your body. Start with 20 to 30 minutes of walking, jogging, swimming, playing tennis or anything else to get your heart rate up. Also, add resistance exercise using lights weights or exercise machines

- Avoid cooking with aluminum-based cookware and consider having your water tested (especially if you use well water) for aluminum.

2-Dietary Tips

- Eat colorful fruits and vegetables that are high in antioxidants and polyphenols (grapes, raspberries, strawberries, spinach, oranges, apples, etc.)

- Drink a cup (or two) of green tea daily, along with your morning coffee (from organic coffee beans of course!)

- If you drink alcohol, drink a glass of red wine with dinner

- Use turmeric to spice up your food

3-Supplements

- Vitamin C: 1,000-2,000 mg/day

- Vitamin D: at least 2,000 I.U./day

- Vitamin E: 400 I.U. units/day (make sure it's a mixed vitamin E with both tocopherols and tocotrienols)

- Resveratrol: 200-400 mg/day

- Vitamin B- complex vitamins (25-50 mg)/ daily, (look for at least 800 mcg of folic acid)

- Fish oil: 2,000-3,000 mg/day

- Alpha-lipoic acid: 200-400 mg/day

- Acetyl-L-carnitine: 1,000 mg/day

- Whey protein: 3-5 grams, 2-3 times a week

- Carnosine: 1,000 mg/day

4-Bioidentical Hormones

If you're over 40, ask your doctor to check your hormone levels. If she or he won't do it or tells you it's a waste of time, get another doctor who knows the vital importance of optimal hormone levels in the fight against chronic diseases.

Chapter 2: Heart Smarts

Quick—what's the single most important part of your body? A lot of people would say it's their heart, and for good reason. This muscle is one of the first organs to be fully formed in an unborn baby. A baby's heartbeat can be heard as early as the sixteenth week of pregnancy. Once your heart starts beating, it continues beating every second of every day for the rest of your life. If you live to be eighty, that comes out to be two and a half billion beats! When your heart stops beating, everything else in your body stops, too.

Cardiovascular disease: public enemy number one

Because a healthy heart is vital to good health, hearing the statistics concerning cardiovascular disease (a blanket term referring to diseases of the heart or blood vessels) can be grim. But I believe that knowledge is power, so here are those scary numbers:

According to figures by the American Heart Association, over 60 million Americans suffer from some form of heart disease, including coronary artery disease, congestive heart failure, and cardiac arrhythmias (abnormal rhythms of the heart). Coronary artery disease alone affects almost 13 million Americans and is the leading cause of death in the United States for both women and men.

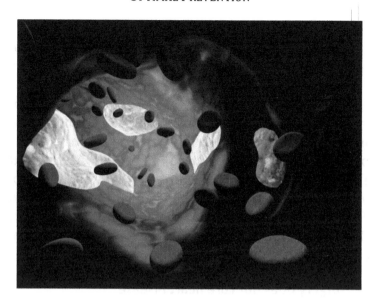

Heart disease isn't just a problem for men

Not too many years ago, physicians thought of heart disease as a man's disease. In fact, many doctors still think heart disease isn't a problem for young and middle-aged women. Yet sadly, heart disease is an equal opportunity killer—out of the approximately 600,000 Americans who will die from heart disease this year, almost 300,000 of them will be a woman. And far too often, women aren't given the same preventive care as men—when they're given any at all—which leads to a lot of unnecessary pain and suffering.

Heart disease: costly in every aspect

Statisticians and politicians often forget that behind every health statistic and dollar is a real live person. It seems easy for them to toss out facts and figures without acknowledging the literal heartache caused by cardiovascular disease, which can steal your ability to enjoy the simple pleasures of life and rob you of your life savings due to lost time at work, visits to doctors and hospitals, and medication costs.

The financial impact of heart disease on health-care costs is staggering, with expenditures running over 200 billion dollars a year. One of the main reasons so much money is spent each year on heart disease is that heart surgery—one of the most expensive surgeries—is a common treatment for heart disease in America. The most common type of surgery for heart disease is a coronary artery bypass graft (CABG, pronounced "cabbage"). Ask around; I'm positive you'll soon find someone who's had this type of heart surgery. Over 300,000 women and men have CABG surgery every year, and the average cost is 45,000 dollars. That yields a tidy sum of 13.5 billion dollars being spent each year for heart surgery!

Heart surgery does not cure heart disease

For $45,000 it might seem reasonable to think that heart surgery can cure heart disease. Unfortunately, it can't. In fact, heart surgery has some potentially serious and life-threatening side effects, such as heart and brain damage. In a study published in the *New England Journal of Medicine*, researchers evaluated over 2,000 patients who had undergone CABG heart surgery. The researchers found that approximately 6% of the patients had developed neurological side effects such as strokes, seizures and deterioration of intellectual functioning.

The messy but necessary details about coronary artery disease

Each year, coronary artery disease takes the lives of over half a million Americans and convinces over 300,000 to have their chests split open for a surgery that may cause brain damage. But just what is this disease? Most doctors believe that, like Alzheimer's, coronary artery disease is a multi-step process that damages the arteries of the heart. Because knowing how heart disease occurs can give you the power to prevent it, I've listed a five-step process that shows what has to happen for you to develop coronary heart disease.

Step 1: Arteries in the heart are injured

<u>Cause</u>

Abnormal elevation of homocysteine (an amino acid found in higher amounts in people with heart disease) and free radicals

<u>Effect</u>

Injury to the innermost layer of arteries throughout the body

Step 2: Inflammation causes further arterial damage

<u>Cause</u>

White blood cells (neutrophils and macrophages)

<u>Effect</u>

Arteries become inflamed and platelets accumulate in the area of arterial injury; blood flow decreases

Step 3: Blood flow slows further

<u>Cause</u>

A build-up of atherosclerotic plaque

<u>Effect</u>

Blood flow in the arteries decreases

Step 4: Inflammation continues

<u>Cause</u>

An increase of bio-chemicals called cytokines

<u>Effect</u>

Inflammation causes further damage to arteries

Step 5: Arteries suffer lasting damage

<u>Cause</u>

Inability of arterial cells to produce nitric oxide

<u>Effect</u>

Blood vessels become hard, then constrict and spasm

What is plaque?

Atherosclerotic plaque (the stuff in your heart, not on your teeth) is a sticky, hard substance that can significantly slow blood flow. Plaque is made up of LDL (low-density lipoprotein) cholesterol. LDL cholesterol is commonly known as "bad" cholesterol because a chemical reaction between LDL cholesterol and free radicals is theorized to lead to the formation of plaque.

AGEs strike again!

Remember AGEs? Well, they're back, and this time they are causing problems not in your head, but in your heart. Groundbreaking research has shown that AGEs are somehow involved in the formation of atherosclerotic plaque.

In a paper published in the *Annals of the New York Academy of Sciences*, researchers examined the role of oxidation and AGEs in the development of atherosclerosis. While it's widely believed that one of the key first steps in the development of coronary artery disease is an inflammatory response in the heart vessel walls, the biochemical changes that lead to this inflammation are still not clear. However, in this paper, researchers showed that a type of AGE (carboxymethyllysine, or CML, for you folks who want to know the details) is formed during times of oxidative stress in the heart and may be involved in the development of atherosclerotic plaques.

Nitric oxide: no laughing matter (at least not for your heart)

If you're thinking nitric oxide is the stuff your dentist gives you before jamming sharp instruments into your mouth, you're almost right: that's nitrous oxide. However, nature has been using nitric oxide much longer than dentists have.

In 1998, the Nobel Prize in Physiology or Medicine was given to three scientists for their research on nitric oxide. It turns out that having adequate levels of nitric oxide in your body is extremely important to good health by regulating shape and function of the cells (called endothelial cells) that line the inside of blood vessels in the heart and throughout the body. If these cells become dysfunctional, they can cause blood vessels to harden, spasm and constrict—three things you certainly don't want your blood vessels doing.

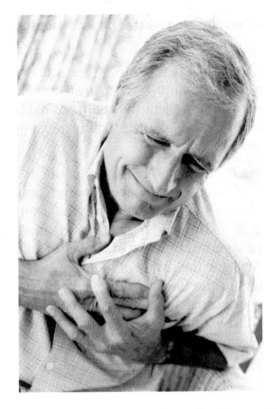

Angina and heart attacks: the end result of heart disease

To help visualize what happens when heart disease causes blockage in the arteries, think of your blood vessels as hoses and your heart as a spigot. If you twist a garden hose when the water is on, you'll cause a blockage and the water will stop flowing out. If you continue to keep the hose blocked, eventually there will either be a tear in the hose or damage back at the spigot.

Similarly, arterial blockage keeps blood from flowing through your arteries to nourish the heart with life-sustaining oxygen. Angina, or chest pain, is one end result of this blockage. A more serious end result is a myocardial infarction, or heart attack. When this happens, a part of your heart can actually die; if enough of your heart dies, so do you.

The big eight and heart attacks

Canadian researchers, through a study of 30,000 people in 52 countries, have identified eight factors that they claim account for at least 90% of all first-time heart attacks, and I find no reason to dispute their findings. In order, the big eight are as follows:

- Smoking
- High cholesterol
- High blood pressure
- Obesity
- Stress
- Lack of exercise
- Diabetes (yes, diabetes is implicated in heart disease as well as Alzheimer's)
- Diet low in fruits and vegetables

How you can and can't prevent heart disease

With approximately half a million American men and women projected to die from heart disease this year alone, it would seem to make perfect sense for prevention of heart disease to be a priority in medicine. At least it makes perfect sense me. Sadly, however, heart disease is still mainly thought of as a condition to be treated rather than aggressively prevented. But prevent it you can, with both conventional and alternative methods.

Before we start, let's note a few hard facts. When I was a teenager, my father told me that it wasn't worth worrying about the things in life you couldn't change, since there were enough things that you could. At the time, I thought that my father didn't know much of anything, but it turns out that my father was right about that. For heart disease, there are a few risk factors you can't change, and therefore should not worry about. Those risk factors are the following:

- Being male
- Being an African-American
- Having type-1 diabetes

Beta-blockers: Old medicines for a 21st century disease

If you're over 50, you might have a bottle of beta-blockers in your medicine cabinet. These commonly prescribed medications reduce blood pressure by slowing the heart rate. As a bonus, studies have shown that beta-blockers can reduce both the symptoms of heart disease and associated deaths. By slowing the heart rate, beta-blockers decrease the oxygen demands of the heart. For people with heart disease, this allows their hearts to better utilize oxygen.

Of course, there's no such thing as a free lunch, and all prescription medications can have unpleasant side effects. Fatigue, lethargy, memory loss and sexual dys-function are some potential side effects of beta-blockers. If you experience these or any other side effects, talk to your doctor about stopping medication. People who abruptly stop taking beta-blockers have been known to experience sudden chest pain and even heart attacks, two things that beta-blockers are supposed to prevent!

Commonly used beta-blockers

Generic name	Brand name
Propranolol	Inderal, InnoPran XL
Atenolol	Tenormin

Generic name	Brand name
Metoprolol	Lopressor, Tropol-XL
Acebutolol	Sectral
Labetalol	Normodyne, Trandate

What causes high blood pressure?

Being diagnosed with high blood pressure—hypertension—is almost a rite of passage for middle-aged and elderly Americans. It's estimated that at least 2 million new cases of high blood pressure will be diagnosed this year in the U.S. alone. Hypertension is called "the silent killer," since it generally produces no major symptoms, while causing widespread damage to your heart and other vital organs. While hypertension can strike at any time, it's most common in older individuals. Among Americans over the age of seventy, 70% of women and 50% of men have hypertension—that comes out to 50 million people!

How high is too high?

Blood pressure is the force of blood against the blood vessels. Blood pressure readings are given as systolic blood pressure over diastolic blood pressure: systolic pressure is your blood pressure as your heart contracts, and diastolic pressure is your blood pressure as your heart relaxes. For many years, guidelines defined normal blood pressure as systolic pressure of 130 or below, and diastolic pressure of 85 or below (130/85). Hypertension was defined as blood pressure at or above 140/90. High normal was defined as anything in between.

A small change is a big deal

At first glance, you might think that having blood pressure 10 or 15 points above normal shouldn't be a big deal. Sometimes you'd be right, as in the case of pregnancy-induced high blood pressure, which only lasts a few months. However, if your blood pressure is elevated for years without any treatment (either conventional or alternative), you will most likely suffer significant damage to many parts of your body, including your heart, your brain and your kidneys. And once the damage is done, there's not a lot you can do about it. So, if you don't want high blood pressure to cause heart disease, kidney failure and impotence (that last one always gets the attention of men), remember the magic word: Prevention!

Aspirin: an oldie but goodie

It has been said that if aspirin were a new drug it would never be available without a prescription. That's because it can do so many things, from treating pain to potentially preventing heart attacks. Studies show that aspirin has a potential role in secondary prevention, although studies on aspirin's role in primary prevention aren't nearly as convincing. Interestingly, the most favorable study on aspirin for primary prevention of heart attacks used Bufferin, which contains a substantial amount of magnesium that has led some innovative researchers to question whether or not it was aspirin or magnesium that worked to prevent heart attacks.

Notwithstanding that controversy, the bottom line is that if you've had a heart attack and your doctor tells you to take an aspirin a day, pay attention. Multiple studies in both women and men have conclusively shown that taking aspirin daily can significantly reduce the chances of having a second heart attack. Unfortunately, it's also known that women, African-Americans, and Hispanics are still less likely to be put on a daily aspirin than men. If you're worried about heart health, ask your doctor if you should be taking aspirin.

ACE inhibitors

Like their beta-blocker older cousins, ACE (angiotensin converting enzyme) inhibitors can lower blood pressure and help prevent hypertension and heart disease. There is now a mass of scientific evidence showing that if you have significant heart disease or have suffered a heart attack, ACE inhibitors can decrease your risk of dying from a second heart attack. A study on over 12,000 men and women reported that patients with heart disease who added an ACE inhibitor to their daily medication regime had a 20% lower risk of dying from a heart attack or a stroke than those who weren't taking an ACE inhibitor. Furthermore, those taking an ACE inhibitor decreased their risk of having a heart attack by 24%. ACE inhibitors are also useful for preventing further heart disease in people who suffer from heart failure as well as diabetes.

The potential side effects of ACE inhibitors (a nagging cough, elevation of blood potassium levels, dizziness and headache) are significantly less severe than those of beta-blockers; however, the effect of ACE inhibitors on the pocketbook can be substantially more painful due to their higher cost. Still, I think that people with early onset heart disease or diabetes should talk to their doc about adding an ACE inhibitor to thcceir daily medication regiment.

Commonly used ACE inhibitors

Generic name	Brand name
Captopril	Capoten
Quinapril	Accupril
Ramipril	Altace
Enalapril	Vasotec
Benazepril	Lotensin

Statins: a cure for heart disease?

You are probably aware that most of the medical community considers hypercholesterolemia, or high cholesterol, a significant contributor to heart disease. Drawing on decades of research, medical researchers state that high levels of cholesterol—or, more specifically, "bad" LDL cholesterol—leads to formation of arterial plaque, or atherosclerosis (number 3 in the five-step heart disease process).

In the late 1990s, researchers conducted large-scale tests of the effects on high LDL cholesterol levels by cholesterol-inhibiting medications known as statins. These studies reportedly showed that when LDL cholesterol levels were lowered through the use of statins, a person could significantly decrease their chance of dying from heart disease. Because of these studies—and a multi-million dollar marketing campaign by pharmaceutical companies—statins are now incredibly popular, though they are not without significant costs.

Statins are quite expensive unless generic forms are available. They also have the potential to cause major side effects, including fatigue, muscle aches and liver damage. Yet despite their potential problems, statins continue to be some of the most widely prescribed medicines in the country.

Are statins a con?

In the medical world, it's almost preached as gospel truth that statins are wonder drugs. Some doctors even advocate giving statins to people who don't have significant heart disease. In fact, when a recent study on 507 people with mild to moderate heart disease showed that high-dose statins reduce heart plaque, some people started thinking that statin drugs may actually be a cure for heart disease.

You may be saying, "A cure for heart disease? That sounds too good to be true." And after reading the study in question, I have to agree—it does sound too good to be true. I say this for two reasons: one, the study was not controlled with a placebo (which is kind of interesting, considering that mainstream practitioners generally throw a fit when studies on supplements or herbs don't use a placebo control); and two, we don't even know if reducing plaque is truly a big deal. Some very reputable doctors think the amount of plaque you have isn't as important as how stable that plaque is.

One of the challenges of twenty-first-century medicine is trying to tease the truth out from studies such as these, especially when drug companies fund the studies. John Abramson, a doctor who has bravely examined the labyrinth of medical research, wrote a book published in 2004 called *Overdosed America* that caused a mild uproar in the medical establishment. In it, Dr. Abramson challenged some of the most cherished "truths" of mainstream medicine, including the mantra of "statins for everyone."

After an exhaustive analysis of all major studies on statins, Abramson came to the following conclusions:

- Men below the age of 65, who have high cholesterol but no significant coronary heart disease, might benefit modestly from taking statins.

- There are no significant studies showing that women below the age of 65 gain any benefit (in terms of preventing heart disease) from statins.

- There are no significant studies showing that men and women over the age of 65 who have high cholesterol levels benefit from taking statins.

An even more recent paper from 2015 lead with the title of "Statins stimulate atherosclerosis and heart failure: pharmacological mechanisms." In it, the authors list in a very logical and concise manner how statins work and conclude that their use very well might be causing coronary artery disease and heart failure.

Pretty wild, eh? Research like this has certainly opened my eyes, and it should open your eyes, too.

Commonly used statin medications

Generic name	Brand name
Lovastatin	Altocor, Mevacor
Fluvastatin	Lescol XL
Atorvastatin	Lipitor
Pravastatin	Pravachol
Simvastatin	Zocor

Complementary and alternative approaches to preventing heart disease

According to recent estimates, Americans spend at least 35 billion dollars a year on vitamins and supplements in their quest to stay healthy. Yet, ask most mainstream doctors about supplements and chances are they'll tell you you're wasting your money. The vast majority of conventionally trained physicians are still skeptical at best and usually disdainful of any treatment that isn't approved by the FDA or promoted by multinational pharmaceutical corporations.

Well, guess what? All those doubting doctors are wrong— dead wrong. Hundreds of credible studies show that numerous vitamins and supplements can help you live longer and fight off deadly chronic health conditions such as heart disease. On the following pages I've picked the best supplements that you should consider now to both prevent and treat heart disease.

Plant Sterols: a Natural Alternative to Statins

You'd be hard-pressed to find a mainstream medical doctor who doesn't think that high cholesterol levels are bad. You'd also be hard-pressed to find a mainstream doctor who knows of any proven alternative therapies to statin medications to lower cholesterol. That's too bad, because there is a safe, natural and effective alternative to statins called plant phytosterols.

So just what are these plant sterols? Interestingly enough, they're in essence plant cholesterol—that is, while we humans make cholesterol, plants make phytosterols. While this might seem strange—taking a plant's "choles- terol" to lower your own cholesterol, there a number of studies showing that phytosterols can significantly lower cholesterol without any of the side effects associated with stains (as always, if you're bored and wish to read hundreds of pages of reference material like I did to write this book, feel free to go to reference section and have at it!). In a nutshell, studies have shown that taking around 2 grams a day of plant sterols can effectively lower your LDL cholesterol by 10-15%. Plant sterols are safe, effective, and inexpensive and are almost always in my recommendations to patients in regards to a heart-healthy supplement regime.

Arginine makes NO a heart-healthy word

Time for a quick test: In the final step of the five-step process of heart disease, what little known, but extremely important, substance helps keep your heart blood vessels soft and pliable? Can't remember? Go ahead and look back; in this test, cheating is not only allowed, it's encouraged!

Did I just hear someone say "nitric oxide?" Give yourself a pat on the back. Nitric oxide (NO) is very important for maintaining your heart's health. NO influences the layer of cells that line the inside of blood vessels in the heart. A lack of NO causes these blood vessels to become dry, brittle and constricted, which can cause a person with heart disease to suddenly have a heart attack. This is no laughing matter. Fortunately, scientists have discovered that the simple, inexpensive supplement arginine (specifically, L-arginine) can help protect against heart disease by increasing the body's production of NO.

One of the first studies on the effects of arginine on heart health was done at the Mayo Clinic in 1998. There, researchers gave patients either nine grams of arginine or a placebo each day. After six months, the patients who had been taking L-arginine had significantly better heart blood flow than did the patients who had been taking placebo. The authors of the study concluded, "Long-term oral L-arginine supplementation for 6 months in humans improves coronary small-vessel endothelial function in association with significant improvements in symptoms and a decrease in plasma endothelial concentrations." In other words, arginine increased the blood flow to the hearts of patients with heart disease, lessening chest pain and other symptoms.

Other studies, done both in Europe and the United States, have shown that arginine can improve heart function in patients with heart disease and a history of angina. In one study researchers gave a short course of L-arginine (six grams a day for three days) to patients with angina and a history of heart attack to see how L-arginine would affect exercise tolerance. Compared to patients who were given a placebo, the patients who were given L-arginine had significant increases in their ability to exercise on a treadmill.

In another study, researchers looked at 42 patients who suffered from angina. The patients were either given 15 grams a day of L-arginine or placebo before exercising on a stationary bicycle. After only 10 days, the patients taking the L-arginine were able to exercise longer and without pain when compared to the patients who were taking placebo. Because of this effect, the authors concluded "L-arginine can be recommended as an [addition] in the treatment of patients with ischemic heart disease."

So much for there being no good studies on alternative medicine, eh? I'm very confident in telling my patients that a daily dose of arginine (5 to 10 grams) is certainly warranted for those who wish to prevent or treat heart disease. And if you aren't interested in doing either, why are you reading this book?

Magnesium can help keep your heart healthy and strong

If you take just one supplement to prevent heart disease, magnesium should be it. This common mineral has been shown in a number of studies to play an important role in preventing or treating a number of cardiovascular illnesses, including the following:

- Atherosclerosis
- Congestive heart disease
- Ischemic heart disease
- Sudden cardiac death
- Cardiac arrhythmias

With an impressive résumé like that, it's no wonder that magnesium is a front-line therapy for heart-disease prevention and a supplement that I recommend to almost all my patients.

B-vitamins, free radicals and heart disease

Let's go all the way back to step one of the five-step process of heart disease, when we learned about the dangers of high levels of homocysteine (an amino acid that is a risk factor for heart disease. Fortunately, you can combat high homocysteine levels through the use of three B-vitamins—vitamin B6, vitamin B12 and folic acid.

A study published in the *JAMA* showed that women who took folic acid and vitamin B6 had a significantly lower occurrence of heart disease when compared to women who had a low intake of folic acid and vitamin B6. Another study in *JAMA* examined the effect of lowering homocysteine levels with vitamin B6, vitamin B12 and folic acid in 553 female and male patients with heart disease. Those patients on the B-vitamin/folic acid regime had significantly fewer symptoms of heart disease—including heart attacks—than those patients who did not take supplements.

Homocysteine isn't the only culprit in the early stages of heart disease. Free radicals also damage your heart and contribute to heart disease. Studies now show that antioxidants such as vitamin C, vitamin E and coenzyme Q10 can help ward off heart disease.

For example, the Nurses' Health study, which examined a population of almost 90,000 female nurses, showed that those who had the highest intake of vitamin E had an astonishing 40% reduction in their risk of developing coronary artery disease. The Cambridge Heart Antioxidant Study showed that vitamin E reduced the risk of non-fatal heart attacks in people with heart disease by 77%.

Other studies have shown that patients with heart disease tend to have lower blood levels of vitamin C. One large study of 11,349 American men and women showed an inverse association between vitamin C intake and death due to heart disease. Finally, a meta-analysis published in Britain on antioxidant vitamin intake and heart disease came to the conclusion that "an increase in dietary intake of antioxidant vitamins has encouraging prospects for possible CHD [heart disease] prevention."

Coenzyme Q10, also known as CoQ10—is touted by some as the miracle supplement of the twenty-first century. Widely available as a supplement, CoQ10 is found in every cell in your body. In addition to its role as an antioxidant, CoQ10 is involved in key biochemical reactions that make energy in your cells. This is worth repeating—without CoQ10, no energy is made in your body. And just like a car won't run without gasoline, your body won't run without energy—without CoQ10, you die.

One way in which CoQ10 can help your heart is by decreasing the oxidation of LDL cholesterol. By doing this, CoQ10 reduces the nasty effects this bad cholesterol can have on the heart. Other studies have shown that CoQ10 supplementation can increase exercise tolerance and decrease chest pain in people with early heart disease. CoQ10 can be useful even for people who have severe heart disease and require CABG surgery: several studies have shown that people who take CoQ10 before surgery have quicker recovery times, less chance of potentially deadly arrhythmias, and stronger hearts.

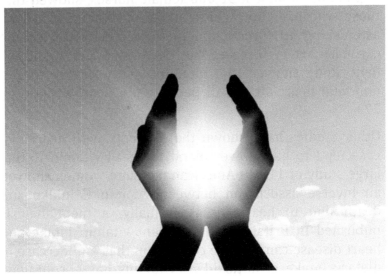

Vitamin D: the sunshine vitamin rises again to help prevent heart disease

So now that you know that vitamin D is vitally important in preventing Alzheimer's, do you really need another reason to take it? If so, consider this (unfortunately) not so well-known fact in the mainstream medical world: vitamin D plays a critical role in warding off heart disease. How do I know this? By studies such as the one in the journal *Current Opinion in Clinical Nutrition and Metabolic Care* linking low vitamin D levels to high blood pressure, inflammation, and sub-clinical vascular disease, all part of the heart disease process. As with Alzheimer's, the potential benefits of vitamin D in preventing heart disease is enormous, yet sadly unknown outside the complementary and integrative medicine world.

Fish Oil: A major player in preventing heart disease

Fish oil is one of the most powerful supplements on the market today in the fight against heart disease. Medical researchers first noticed the heart-protective potential of fish oil when they looked at the Inuit, the native people populating Alaska and northern Canada. A significant part (and at times of the year, the only part) of the Inuit's diet is salmon, which is high in omega-3 fatty acids, specifically eicosapentaenoic acid (EPA) and docosahexaenoic acid (DHA). Now you might think, "Hey, if all they're eating is fat, they're probably having heart attacks left and right!" Well, guess what—the Inuit have a very low incidence of heart disease and sudden cardiac death. Researchers now believe that the number one reason for this low rate of heart disease among the Inuit is their consumption of omega-3 fatty acids.

Since the mid-1990s, study after study has shown that both women and men who have a high intake of omega-3 fatty acids have much less risk of developing heart disease or dying from a heart attack. For people who already have heart disease or have already had a heart attack, omega-3 fatty acids can slow the disease's progression and decrease the chance of a second heart attack. There is even some evidence that fish oil supplements decrease the risk of atherosclerotic lesions redeveloping in people who have had CABG surgery.

One of the most deadly effects of heart disease is the risk of sudden cardiac death. It has been estimated that sudden cardiac death accounts for at least 50% of all deaths attributed to heart disease. The majority of these deaths are thought to be caused by the heart going into an arrhythmia, a condition in which the heart beats in an irregular, uncoordinated fashion; the heart is still beating, but no blood is being pumped.

While many common prescription medications and surgical interventions are used to help prevent cardiac arrhythmias, there is no evidence that any of these therapies work. However, there is now solid evidence that omega-3 fatty acids in fish oils may substantially reduce the risk of deadly cardiac arrhythmias, proving once again that the wisdom of our elders is not something to brush away in our sophisticated, technologically advanced twenty-first century. If you don't like eating fish every day, two grams of a fish oil supplement can give you the same protection as a hunk of salmon.

Supplements to help cool the inflammation

The next time you go see a doctor—especially one who practices integrative medicine—they may order a blood test looking at your levels of C-reactive protein, or CRP. Integrative doctors like myself routinely test for this protein because it can give us a good idea about your levels of inflammation. I hope you are thinking "hey, didn't you talk about inflammation being part of the process of heart disease?"

I did. Inflammation occurs in steps two and four of the five-part process of coronary artery disease. Lower levels of C-reactive protein suggest a lower chance of having another heart attack if you've had one already. Even if you have otherwise normal levels of cholesterol, high levels of CRP can help predict if you're still at higher risk of developing heart disease. Pretty nifty, eh?

For those of you looking for natural ways to maintain optimal health, the good news is that exciting new research shows that vitamins and supplements can naturally and safely decrease your CRP levels. Studies have shown that people who take vitamin E, vitamin B6 and antioxidants such as vitamin C and selenium have lower (healthier) CRP levels.

Vitamin C: Was Linus Pauling right?

Want another way to get your mainstream medical doctor all cranked up? Ask them about the work of Linus Pauling, the Nobel Prize-winning scientist (and in my opinion, one of the greatest minds of the twentieth century) who said the low levels of vitamin C were associated with a number of chronic diseases, including cancer and heart disease. Most mainstream docs dismiss Pauling's work with a dismissive wave of their hand, yet if they take the time like I have to read his research on vitamin C and chronic disease, they'll find a very compelling argument.

In a nutshell, what Pauling said was this: humans (and interestingly enough, guinea pigs) cannot synthesize vitamin C, so we must get it from our diets. However, in our distant past, our consumption of vitamin C-containing foods (mainly fruits and vegetables) was much higher than it is today. While many people may only get 100 milligrams or so of vitamin C in their diet, Pauling hypothesized that we need much more—3,000, 5,000, even 10,000 milligrams daily—to ward off chronic diseases such as heart disease. Even more heretical, he theorized that high levels of vitamin C could actually reverse heart disease!

Dr. Pauling was a brilliant pioneer and his ideas deserve to be looked into in detail. Unfortunately, since the profit margin for vitamin C is insignificant, that work just isn't being done and probably won't be done for the foreseeable future. However, that doesn't mean you can't be proactive and take in enough vitamin C—either through diet or supplements—to help protect against the chronic medical problems like heart disease that are killing millions of us every year.

The link between hormones and heart disease

In the last chapter, I showed you how having optimal hormone levels could protect you against Alzheimer's. But the news keeps getting better: not only can hormones protect your brain from falling apart, but they can also protect you from heart disease.

In the past 15-20 years, the research on healthy hormone levels has gone through the roof, and we now know that maintaining optimal hormone levels not only keeps us functioning sexually, it significantly lessens our odds of developing debilitating chronic diseases such as Alzheimer's and heart disease. Yet like so many other medical issues, people who espouse the rational use of bio-identical hormones are termed quacks or worse. For instance, the actress Suzanne Somers has been vilified for her enthusiasm for bio-identical hormones and supplements, yet anyone who knows anything about medicine will find her books to be fascinating and illuminating reads.

So let's talk about hormones and heart disease. With regards to men, multiple studies have shown that men who have low testosterone levels are at high risk for heart disease. For example, a study out of Norway—The Tromso Study—followed over 1,500 hundred men over an eleven-year period and showed conclusively that men who had the lowest levels of free testosterone had a 24% increase of death from heart disease.

For women, the data is just as compelling. A great review article in the journal *Postgraduate Medicine*, clearly cited multiple studies that showed bio-identical (not synthetic) estrogen and progesterone decreased LDL cholesterol levels, increased HDL cholesterol levels, and reduced coronary artery spasm (which is known to increase a woman's risk of heart attack and stroke). The bottom line here is clear: to help prevent heart disease, keep track of your hormones as you age. Then, if you and your doctor decide hormone replacement therapy is in order, keep your hormones at healthy levels through the use of bio-identical—not synthetic—hormones.

Behavioral changes to prevent heart disease

All of us, rich or poor, male or female, old or young, live in a quick-fix world. Who among us doesn't look for the answers to life's questions that require the least amount of time while promising the biggest return?

Health care certainly doesn't escape these unrealistic expectations. Multinational pharmaceutical corporations spend hundreds of millions a dollars a year advertising the quick and painless ways that their medications can alleviate everything from hemorrhoids to heart attacks. However, it's a wise person that remembers there are generally no quick fixes in medicine, at least not for chronic conditions such as heart disease. You can be on all the expensive medications in the world and take the most cutting edge supplements on the market, yet if you engage in certain deleterious behaviors, no medication or supplement will matter.

As human beings, we were made to be active and to follow a certain type of healthy diet. Unfortunately, those of us living in this technologically advanced world generally do the exact opposite, and our health suffers because of it. In the following section I've listed some sensible—and certainly doable—behavioral changes that will not only help you prevent heart disease, but will also help you feel better and live a longer, healthier life.

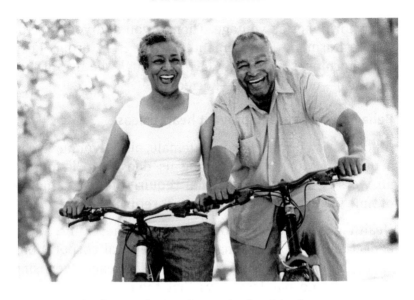

Exercise: the key to longevity and a healthy heart

Our bodies aren't made to sit at a desk for eight hours a day in front of a computer screen, then drive home and sit on the couch in front of the TV for three hours. To maintain proper health, especially heart health, some type—any type—of exercise must be part of your life.

Multiple studies have looked at the effects of exercise on heart disease in people both young and old, and the results consistently show that exercise can help prevent heart disease (while warding off osteoporosis and obesity). In the Women's Health Study, researchers followed 40,417 postmenopausal women with an average age of 62 for seven years. Quite simply, those women who exercised more had less heart disease. Another similar study showed that elderly men who walked or bicycled for 20 minutes at least three times a week had a significant 30% reduction in their risk for developing and dying from heart disease.

The message from these and numerous other studies is clear: getting off your behind and doing something you enjoy—be it walking, bicycling, swimming or any activity that gets your heart rate up for 15 to 20 minutes a few times a week—can truly be a life saver.

Stress kills

Have you ever known anybody who seemed to wither away—or maybe even died—when faced with an over-whelmingly stressful situation like the death of a loved one? While most people instinctively know that stress is bad for you, it's only been in the past few years that mainstream medicine has acknowledged this ancient truth.

A growing body of scientific evidence now shows that stress brought on by job unhappiness, social isolation and feelings of hopelessness is an independent risk factor for the development of heart disease and heat attacks. Fortu-nately, there is some good news: studies have also shown that stress-management training for people with high levels of stress reduces the risk of heart attacks by 74%. The take-home message is that by reducing your stress levels (through yoga, meditation, exercise, golf or what-ever else you consider relaxing), you'll be doing your heart and your overall health a great deal of good.

Cigarettes and heart disease: two deadly friends

In my opinion, the greatest positive change over the past 30 years has been the mainstream medical community's realization of the dangers of smoking, especially in terms of cancer and heart disease. Is it really a surprise to anyone in twenty-first-century America that cigarettes are a significant health hazard? Is there anyone out there who doesn't believe that cigarettes directly contribute to such wonderful things as heart disease, cancer and impotence? Such persons should contact their local 'flat earth society'—I hear they're in need of new recruits.

That cigarette smoking is a major contributor to the development of heart disease is old news. Very few people are surprised to hear that smokers have a heart attack rate five times higher than that of nonsmokers, or that cigarette smoking is directly responsible for at least 20% of all deaths from heart disease (which comes out to around 120,000 deaths a year). Smoking just one cigarette causes platelets to become stickier and arteries to spasm, two events directly related to heart attacks.

I know it's not easy to quit smoking; I tried four or five times before I gave the habit up. (I'm many things, but I'm not a hypocrite—I couldn't counsel my patients to give up their smokes if I was still puffing away myself!) But if you want to do just one thing to significantly decrease your risk of heart disease, then stop smoking!

When you finally decide to quit smoking, remember that for many people, quitting is a process, not a one-time event. If you don't succeed the first time, try again. By looking at smoking cessation as a series of gradual steps that might have to be repeated more than once, you will be more able to understand, control, and eventually kick your smoking habit.

The many benefits of quitting smoking

It's never too late to quit smoking. If you quit now, your body will immediately start becoming healthier in the following ways:

- 20 minutes after quitting: your heart rate begins to decline, lowering your blood pressure

- 12 hours after quitting: the level of carbon monoxide (a deadly, colorless gas also found in auto exhaust) drops to normal

- 2-4 weeks after quitting: your lungs begin to clear themselves and your heart attack risk starts to decrease

- 3 months after quitting: your lung capacity begins to noticeably improve and that annoying smoker's cough disappears

- 1 year after quitting: your risk of CAD is now half that of smokers

- 5 years after quitting: your risk of having a stroke is reduced to that of a non-smoker

- 10 years after quitting: your lung cancer risk is half that of a smoker

- 15 years after quitting: your risk of CAD is back to that of a non-smoker

Dietary changes: healthy foods for a happy heart

During the last 30 years, both mainstream medical organizations and the U.S. government have officially sanctioned (and spent millions of your hard-earned tax dollars promoting) a low-fat, high-carbohydrate diet. During that same time, there has been an explosion of obesity, diabetes and heart disease in this country. What a coincidence! The sad fact is that eating a lot of carbohydrate-rich foods (such as pasta and bread) and passing over so-called fatty foods is a sure path to bad health. Fats, as you've learned by now, aren't necessarily bad for you, and certain ones, like omega-3 fatty acids, are essential for optimal health.

Good fats vs. bad fats

When people talk about good fats and bad fats, they're referring to saturated fats and unsaturated fats. Saturated fats, such as those found in margarine, butter and beef, are solid at room temperature. These saturated fats, which are quite prevalent in our modern fast-food diet, are thought to be major factors in many conditions such as heart disease and cancer. Other studies have refuted this. Until more definitive studies are done, eating foods with a moderate amount of saturated fats shouldn't be frowned upon. In contrast to saturated fats are monounsaturated and polyunsaturated fats. These fats are generally very soft or even liquid at room temperature. More and more research indicates that both of these fats are essential to good health. Common sources of monounsaturated fats include olive oil and peanut oil. Polyunsaturated fats are found in sunflower oil, corn oil, flaxseed oil, and fish oil.

Trans-fatty acids: the Frankenstein's monster of fats

Both saturated and unsaturated fats are natural—that is, they're found in the foods we've eaten ever since humans started walking on the earth. However, a portion of the fat intake of Americans, especially those who love fast food, is made up of a fat created in the laboratory.

Trans-fatty acids (trans fats) are made by chemically changing polyunsaturated fats, which degrade rapidly and have a short shelf life, into a more stable fat that does not spoil as quickly. Because of their stability, trans fats are found in many fast foods such as cookies, potato chips, and most other baked goods. The problem is that our bodies have not evolved to use these fats. There is now disturbing evidence that people with diets high in trans fats have a significantly increased risk of heart disease, and perhaps even cancer.

If there's one type of fat to avoid, it's this one. The FDA has mandated that manufacturers list the amount of trans fatty acids on food labels, so learn to be a savvy shopper and avoid these heart-clogging synthetic fats.

Eat your fruits, vegetables and whole grains

An article in *JAMA* gave a nice review of major dietary factors that can help prevent heart disease. What the authors found was what most people already know, yet often find hard to do. In the authors' own words,

Substantial evidence indicates that diets using non-hydrogenated unsaturated fats [diets that avoid trans-fatty acids] as the predominate form of dietary fat, whole grains as the main form of carbohydrates, an abundance of fruits and vegetables, and adequate omega-3 fatty acids, can offer significant protection against CHD (coronary heart disease). Such diets... may prevent the majority of cardiovascular diseases in Western populations.

(What, you want a translation in English? Okay, here it is—eat a diet high in fruits and vegetables and push away the triple-decker cheeseburgers!)

How to eat a healthy diet

Choice is a good thing. However, being presented with the overwhelming array of foods at your local supermarket may actually make it difficult for you to pick out the healthiest of foods. To help you make wise choices, I offer the following heart-healthy suggestions for breakfast, lunch and dinner.

- Breakfast: Whole grain breads, bagels, cereals or oatmeal with crushed walnuts or almonds; a hard-boiled egg; organic yogurt, cottage cheese and soymilk; choice of fruits, especially bananas, apricots, strawberries and oranges.

- Lunch: Whole grain English muffin, pita bread or bagel; legumes, such as kidney beans, peas and lentils; choice of at least two vegetables, especially tomatoes, carrots, squash or broccoli; choice of at least one to two fruits.

- Dinner: Lean organic meat or fish; at least two vegetables, including turnip greens, cauliflower, sweet potatoes and artichokes; choice of at least two fruits; red wine (Pinot Noir, Cabernet Sauvignon or Merlot).

Heart-healthy foods

Foods	Nutrients	Effects
Bananas, nuts, whole grain	B-Vitamins	decrease homocysteine level
Fish, nuts, spinach, wheat germ	CoQ-10	antioxidant, energy producer
Almonds, peanuts, spinach, tofu	Magnesium	Energy producer, decrease blood pressure
Fish (salmon, sardines, mackerel), flax seeds	Omega-3 fatty acids	reduces inflammation, decreases risk of sudden cardiac death
Citrus fruits, broccoli, spinach, cauliflower, tomatoes	Vitamin C	Antioxidant, increases blood vessel flexibility
Almonds, whole grains, brown rice	Vitamin E	Antioxidant, decreases blood clotting

Can a glass of wine a day really keep a heart attack away?

Two or three times a year the media reports that alcohol is good for you. These reports provide fodder for late-night talk show jokes and spawn heated debates about the role of alcohol in a person's health.

A number of sound studies have shown that one or two drinks (for our purposes, one drink consists of a beer, a glass of wine or a shot of hard liquor) a day can reduce your overall risk of heart disease. At a meeting of the American Society of Hypertension, researchers reported on a study of 243 European women and men between the ages of 15 and 80 who had one drink a day of beer, wine or hard liquor. The study showed that these moderate drinkers, regardless of age or sex, had significantly better elasticity of their arteries, which translates into better cardiovascular health. Another study reported in *The New England Journal of Medicine* followed over 38 thousand male health professionals for 12 years. The results showed that the men who drank alcohol three or more times a week had a reduced risk of having a heart attack.

In addition to improving heart blood vessel health and reducing your risk of having a heart attack, wine contains polyphenols (remember those?), which are thought to provide heart protection by reducing the risk of blood clots. From the favorable studies now in, it seems reasonable to suggest that if you enjoy a beer during a hot summer day or like to have a glass of wine with a meal of Brussels sprouts and salmon, then by all means do so.

You can prevent heart disease!

A heart attack can strike quickly and forcefully, stealing your life just when you thought you could slow down and enjoy the fruits of a lifetime of hard work. Heart disease will kill over 100,000 Americans this year and take away the simple pleasures of life from hundreds of thousands more. If you don't want to become part of these grim statistics, then you need to start thinking about prevention now. Follow the steps presented in this chapter and work with your integrative medicine physician to tailor a heart disease prevention program—for your own sake, and for the sake of your loved ones.

Strategies to prevent heart disease

Behavioral Tips

- Exercise 20 to 30 minutes at least every other day
- Stop smoking (but you already knew that, right?)
- Eat a diet high in fruits, vegetables and legumes, along with a daily glass of red wine (if you're so inclined)
- Practice stress reduction—yoga, meditation, sex (which for some people will also count as exercise!)

Medications

- Beta-blockers
- Aspirin
- ACE inhibitors
- Cholesterol-lowering medications (statins)

Supplements

- Plant Sterols: 2 grams/day
- Arginine: 2-4 g/day
- Magnesium: 400-800 mg/day
- B-vitamin complex: 25-50 mg/day
- Folic acid: 400-800 mcg/day
- Vitamin C: 1,000-2,000 mg/day
- Vitamin D: 2,000-4,000 I.U. daily
- Vitamin E (as mixed tocopherols/tocotrienols): 200-400 IU/day
- Coenzyme Q10: 100-200 mg/day
- Fish oil (omega-3 fatty acids): 2-4 g/day

Chapter 3: Cerebrovascular Disease: Preventing the Great Disabler

Pop quiz time: What's the leading cause of disability in the United States and the third leading cause of death? You might think car accidents, but the answer is strokes. Cerebrovascular disease, or strokes, afflict 800,000 Americans each year; on the average, someone in the U.S. suffers a stroke every minute, while every 105 seconds someone dies of a stroke. In terms of health-care costs (and just what politician these days doesn't love to tell how they're going to control costs without ever telling us how?), it's estimated that costs related to strokes will be about 63 billion dollars this year. Yet for some reason, prevention of cerebrovascular disease is almost non-existent in the minds of those who control the financial resources of our medical community. And that's a crying shame.

Think that just because you're young you don't have to worry about having a stroke? Unfortunately, you need to think again. Researchers at a American Stroke Association Conference presented data showing that that incidence of strokes among young and middle-aged Americans is rising at a frightening rate. Comparing rates of hospitalizations for strokes between 1994-1995 and 2006-2007, researchers showed that there was a 51% increase in strokes among men aged 15-34 and a 47% increase in men aged 35-44. In women, the numbers were lower but still alarming: among women aged 15-34, rates went up 17% vs. an increase in 36% among women aged 35-44.

So what's causing this increase? As of now, there's no definitive answer, but all signs point to the increase in obesity, high blood pressure, and other risk factors that feed the risks of having a stroke in the first place.

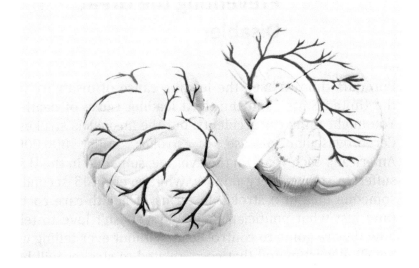

What are strokes?

In simple terms, a stroke is when your brain doesn't get the oxygen it needs (and the brain needs a lot—it's the single biggest user of oxygen in your body) due to a problem in the blood vessels that supplies oxygen to your brain. There are different types of strokes, and it is worth a few minutes of your time to learn them since certain preventive measures don't cover them all. Therefore, without further ado, here's your list.

1. Ischemic strokes

Ischemic strokes happen when a blood vessel that supplies oxygen to your brain becomes clogged or blocked. When this happens, your brain doesn't get oxygen and brain cells quickly begin to die off. Most strokes (around

80%) fall into this category. Ischemic strokes are further subdivided into two more categories: **thrombotic strokes**, which are caused by a blood clot inside your brain, and embolic strokes, which are caused by blood clots that start somewhere else and then travel to your brain. Thrombotic strokes often occur in the elderly and in people who have significant atherosclerosis; **embolic strokes** can occur in people who have recently had surgery or have atrial fibrillation (a condition in which a part of the heart isn't beating properly).

2. Hemorrhagic strokes

Hemorrhagic strokes occur when blood vessels in the brain burst. When this happens, not only does the part of the brain supplied by the broken blood vessel become starved for oxygen, the blood from the ruptured blood vessel causes pressure to build up inside the brain, which can cause even more brain damage. Hemorrhagic strokes also come in two varieties: **intracerebral hemorrhagic strokes**, in which the broken blood vessels are directly inside the brain, and **subarachnoid hemorrhagic strokes**, in which bleeding occurs in the subarachnoid space (between the brain and the membranes that cover the brain). Intracerebral strokes are usually caused by untreated high blood pressure and can occur very rapidly. Subarachnoid strokes often occur due to aneurysms (a weak area of a blood vessel) or an arteriovenous malformation (AVM), a congenital disorder in which a person is born with a weakened tangle of arteries and veins.

Are there such things as mini-strokes?

You may have heard of someone having what they referred to as a mini-stroke. These mini-strokes (or, as they're called in medicine, transient ischemic attacks [TIA]) do happen and are extremely important predictors of having a major stroke. Like ischemic strokes, TIAs are caused by the lack of blood flow to the brain. However, unlike ischemic strokes, TIAs last only seconds to minutes and cause no lasting damage. If you think you've had a TIA, get to your doctor now—studies show us that people who've had TIAs are at higher risk for having a major stroke in the following days, weeks or months.

How can I tell if I'm having a stroke?

Most people who have a stroke or TIA know that something is wrong. If you start experiencing any of the following symptoms, do not wait, do not pass go, don't "just wait and see what happens"—call 911!

- Sudden severe headache (patients with headaches caused by an ischemic stroke will often state that "this is the worst headache of my life")

- Sudden vision loss or significant visual changes

- Sudden dizziness

- Sudden loss of coordination or balance

- Sudden mental confusion or difficulty speaking or understanding speech (men, this does not include suddenly not understanding your wife when she asks you to fix the sink in the middle of the World Series)

- Sudden numbness or weakness on one (or both) sides of your body

The known risk factors for strokes

We know about several risk factors for both ischemic and hemorrhagic strokes: some you can control, others you can't. According to the American Heart Association, the following are risk factors for strokes that none of us have any control over:

- Age: the risk of strokes doubles for each decade after the age of 55.

- Sex: Strokes are more common in men than women. However, it's worth remembering that more than half the deaths caused by strokes are female.

- Race: Strokes are significantly more common in African-Americans than in Caucasians.

- Heredity: A significant part of our health is determined by genetics—if your grandmother or father or brother had a stroke, you are at higher risk of having a stroke.

At this point, you might be thinking, "Hey, doc, why are you telling me about these risk factors? There's not a thing I can do about any of them!" That's true, but you still need to know about them; if they apply to you, then you need to pay extra attention to the following stroke risk factors that you can control.

- **High blood pressure**: Having uncontrolled high blood pressure is the number one controllable risk factor for strokes. If you have high blood pressure, go back to the second chapter and re-read the section on hypertension.

- **Smoking**: Any surprise here? I thought not. If you smoke, not only do you put yourself at higher risk for heart attacks, cancer and Alzheimer's, you also increase your chance of having a stroke. If you're a woman who's on birth control pills (which also increases your risk for a stroke) and you smoke, then you are significantly increasing your risk for having a stroke.

- **Diabetes**: Diabetes is another controllable risk factor for strokes. (If you just can't wait to find out how to prevent diabetes, feel free to jump to Chapter 4—I won't mind!)

- **Heart disease**: Starting to see a common thread? You should, since today's modern epidemics such as heart disease, diabetes, and strokes all work together to rob you of a long, healthy life. In my practice it's quite rare to see a patient with just heart disease or just diabetes—generally, if you've got one, you've got something else too.

You can prevent strokes!

In putting this book together, I strongly considered putting information about strokes in with the chapter on heart disease. While I decided that the information on strokes was important enough to merit its own chapter, that doesn't mean that strokes aren't intimately connected to heart disease.

For one, heart disease and strokes share several risk factors, like elevated cholesterol levels, high blood pressure and smoking. In addition, having coronary heart disease is itself a risk factor for strokes. The bottom line is that some of the preventive measures for heart disease from the last chapter can also help protect you from being one of the 800,000 Americans who will have a stroke this year.

While heart disease and strokes share common features, there's a whole lot of information out there specifically on preventing strokes. Unfortunately, it's not common knowledge to most doctors, who have to spend far too much time dealing with insurance companies, HMOs, and government regulators rather than dig through mountains of research. But don't fret, because I've done most of the work for you and your doctor!

Exercise: a workout for every ill, including strokes

As you read through this book you'll notice I'm unequivocally in favor of exercise, and for good reason—regular exercise has been shown to provide a myriad of benefits, including a decreased risk of having a stroke. A review article in the prestigious journal *Stroke*, examined 23 studies on the benefits of exercise. What these 23 studies showed was irrefutable: men and women who engaged in moderate to high levels of physical exercise significantly decreased their risk of both ischemic and hemorrhagic strokes. Instead of frying your brain cells with the television, get off the couch for a daily dose of physical activity; it's some of the best medicine I know of.

What you eat affects more than just your waistline

Remember the diet I outlined in the last chapter that was loaded with fruits and vegetables? Research has shown that not only can this diet help you prevent heart disease—it also helps you prevent strokes. A study from Denmark looked at over 54,000 men and women and showed that a diet high in fruits significantly decreased the risk of an ischemic stroke.

An even larger study—this one looking at over 71,000 women who ranged in age from 38 to 63 years—showed that the typical American diet loaded with red meat (that double-decker hamburger for lunch), refined grains (the bun on which those hamburger patties sit) and sweets (that chocolate shake to top it all off) puts you at a significantly higher risk for all types of strokes. Moreover, the study also showed that diets high in fruits, vegetables, fish and whole grains could protect against strokes.

Fish oil to the rescue!

You might be thinking to yourself "Dr. Rosick, aren't you talking about the same things over and over again each chapter?" I guess you could think of it that way—certainly supplements like fish oil are useful in preventing a number of chronic diseases—but since these supplements

ARE so important I think it's worth detailing them where they can do the most good.

Okay, onto more fish oil stuff. The idea that fish consumption—and hence, fish oil consumption—can lead to a decreased risk of strokes isn't new. An early study done in1994 on 552 men between age 50 and 69 in the Netherlands showed that those who regularly ate fish had a statistically decreased risk of strokes. However, the studies that convinced the mainstream medical community that omega-3 fatty acids had a role in preventing strokes were published in *JAMA* nearly 10 years later.

The first of these studies examined data from over 79,000 women over a 14-year period; during this time, the women who had the highest intake of fish high in omega-3 fatty acids had significantly decreased risk of strokes, especially thrombotic strokes. The next of these studies looked at data from over 43,000 men over a 12-year period. This study showed that men who ate more fish high in omega-3 fatty acids significantly decreased their risk of ischemic strokes. Other studies have looked at the association between omega-3 fatty acids and health in the elderly, with the same results: people who eat fish high in omega-3 fatty acids lower their risk of strokes. Can it get any plainer than that?

Green tea: a simple yet powerful stroke fighter

Since most green tea in the world is consumed in Asia—specifically Japan and China—it makes sense that most of the research on the health benefits of green tea comes from that region. One Japanese study examined the effects of green tea on strokes in almost 6,000 women aged 40 and older. The results showed that the incidence of strokes was 5.5 times higher in women who drank no green tea than it was in women who drank green tea daily. A study in China examined 14,212 men and women aged 35 to 60 and found that those who drank green tea daily had a significant decrease in their risk of strokes. While it's not yet known how green tea protects against strokes, that's no reason for you not to add this tasty beverage to your daily diet and decrease your risk of becoming another stroke victim.

Coffee can do more than just give you a morning pick-me-up

"What if I'm not a tea drinker?" I can hear some of you say. "What if I just can't do without my cup (or two) of coffee every day?" If you're one of those people (and I certainly am—not that I don't like green tea, but it's certainly no substitute for a good cup of morning coffee) don't fret—a study published in the prestigious journal *Stroke* has shown that, at least for women, coffee can reduce the risk of ischemic strokes.

The particulars for the study were very promising: Out of the 34,670 women—aged 49-83—who drank one or more cups of coffee a day there was a 22-25% lower risk of strokes then in women who didn't drink coffee.

"But I'm not a woman," my male readers will say. "Will coffee lower my risk of having a stroke?" The most we can say right now is "maybe." After all, coffee is a known anti-oxidant and reduces overall inflammation, two factors that are part of the stroke cascade. Being an optimist, I'm going to keep having my cup (or two) of coffee a day and know that not only am I keeping my brain awake, I'm also probably protecting it against the ravages of a stroke.

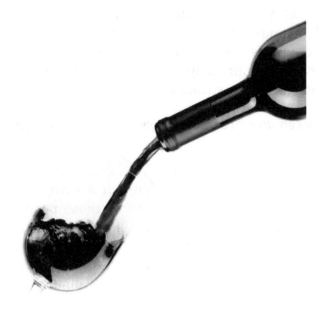

Can a glass of wine a day keep strokes away?

In the first two chapters, I presented some studies that show how a daily glass or two of wine may prevent Alzheimer's disease and heart disease. A reasonable person might ask, "If that's so, can a daily glass or two of wine also prevent me from having a stroke?" Judging from the data now available, I'd say yes.

I base this answer on a couple of studies. In the first one by the American Heart Association, researchers followed over 13,000 men and women age 45 to 84 for 16 years. During that time, 833 strokes were recorded among the group. The researchers found that men and women who drank a moderate amount of wine (approximately one to two glasses a day) had a decreased risk of strokes when compared to those who didn't drink any. However, the researchers noted no decrease in stroke risk for people who drank other types of liquor (such as beer or whiskey).

Another study, done on over 38,000 men, confirmed these findings and showed that while men who drank red wine decreased their risk of strokes, those who drank other alcoholic beverages did not; in fact, heavy drinkers (three or more drinks a day) actually increased their risk of strokes. The bottom line here is simple: if you're going to drink, have no more than two drinks a day. If you're a red wine drinker, take heart in knowing that you're protecting yourself against dementia, heart attacks and strokes!

Can an apple a day keep strokes away?

"An apple a day keeps the doctor away." How many times have you heard that? While some old sayings hold no truth to them, this one does... especially when it comes to strokes. In one study, researchers looked at the incidence of strokes in 552 men, age 50 to 69, who ate a diet high in fruits and vegetables. The researchers found that those men who had a high intake of an antioxidant called quercetin had a lower risk of strokes.

Since apples are high in quercetin, a 28-year study of 9,208 Finnish men and women looked at apple and quercetin intake and stroke risk. However, this study showed that while men and women who had a high consumption of apples had a significant decrease in strokes, it wasn't—at least according to these authors— the quercetin that led to this decrease.

Confused? Don't be. Science is, at best, inexact. And really, in order for it to be useful, it doesn't always have to be exact. Just know that a diet high in fruits—especially apples—can help keep strokes away!

Vitamin D: The fighter of all chronic diseases?

As I researched this book, the research on vitamin D almost overwhelmed me. It's use in preventing all the major chronic diseases—Alzheimer's, heart disease, strokes, diabetes, and cancer—is there for the world to see. Yet when was the last time you heard the government extolling us to get our vitamin D blood levels checked or take vitamin D supplements?

So as with Alzheimer's and heart disease, having optimal vitamin D is critically important in preventing strokes. A study in the journal *Stroke* compared the levels of vitamin D in the blood of stroke victims to the levels of vitamin D levels in otherwise healthy people. The researchers found that vitamin D levels were low in 77% of the stroke victims.

Does this mean that low vitamin D levels can cause strokes? We don't know; however, we do know that vitamin D is involved in a multiple of vitally important bodily functions, so have your doctor check your vitamin D levels, and if you're low, take a vitamin D supplement. Disease prevention doesn't get any easier than that!

Antioxidants: are they useful for preventing strokes?

There are dozens of well-designed studies showing that supplemental antioxidants help prevent a number of chronic diseases, including strokes. One early study published in 1997 showed that vitamin C and beta-carotene—two widely used antioxidants—might play a role in stroke prevention. Researchers looked at the role of vitamin C and beta-carotene in preventing strokes among 1,843 men and found that men taking high doses of vitamin C and beta-carotene had lower rates of strokes than men who took didn't take any vitamin supplements.

A more recent study showed that supplemental antioxidants—specifically, vitamin C and vitamin E—decreased the risk of strokes. Finally, an even more recent study looked at the blood levels of carotenoid antioxidants (specifically, alpha-carotene, beta-carotene and lycopene) and vitamin E in almost 15,000 men over a period of 13 years. Not surprisingly, the researchers found that the men who had the highest blood levels of carotenoids (but, interestingly enough, not vitamin E) had the lowest risk of ischemic strokes.

You might be asking, "Are you saying that I should take antioxidants for stroke prevention or not?" I'd prefer that everyone—myself included—get all their vitamins, including antioxidants, from fruits and vegetables. However, I'm a realist and I recognize that the chances of that happening for even the most health-conscious person are slim to none. Therefore, I think it's reasonable to take a quality multi-vitamin, multi-mineral supplement with all the essential antioxidants such as vitamin C, E, and carotenoids.

Folic acid: good for pregnant women, good for preventing strokes

You may be familiar with folic acid from news reports touting its effects in preventing neural tube defects in developing fetuses. However, folic acid is useful for preventing other serious diseases, including strokes. An article in the prestigious medical journal *The Lancet* looked at eight randomized controlled studies (with a total of 16,841 subjects, male and female) that examined the effects of folic acid on stroke prevention. This meta-analysis showed that supplemental folic acid significantly reduced the risk of strokes. Considering these results, I see no reason for doctors not to recommend supplemental folic acid for the primary prevention of strokes.

Low Testosterone in Men = Higher risk for Strokes

So up until know I've told you that having optimal hormone levels can help prevent Alzheimer's and heart disease. Now I'm about to tell you that in men, having low testosterone levels increases the risk of strokes and TIAs.

An article in the *Journal of Clinical Endocrinology Metabolism* clearly marked the relationship between testosterone levels in elderly men and the risk of stroke. In this study—a prospective observational study of over 3,000 men—researchers showed that in elderly men, the lower the testosterone level the higher the risk for stroke or TIA. Even men who had low normal levels had an increased risk. Therefore, as with Alzheimer's and heart disease, it behooves men to have their testosterone levels checked on a yearly basis, just as we do with other things like cholesterol and blood sugar levels. If it's low—even low normal—then find yourself a physician who's well versed in hormonal replacement therapy and start decreasing your chances of stroking out!

The time to prevent strokes is now!

As a physician trained in preventive medicine, it's heartbreaking for me to see patients who have diseases or conditions like strokes that very well could have been prevented. To be cut down by a stroke in your golden years—the period of life you should be able to enjoy after decades of hard work—is something that none of us want to face. Talk to your doctor about the recommendations below, and begin these steps today to prevent strokes.

Strategies to prevent strokes

<u>**Behavioral Tips**</u>

- Exercise 20 to 30 minutes at least every other day

- Stop smoking (You can never hear this enough!)

- Eat a diet high in fruits, vegetables, and whole grains, along with daily glasses of red wine and green tea

<u>Medications</u> to help prevent strokes

- ACE inhibitors
- Aspirin
- Beta-blockers

<u>Supplements</u>

- Folic acid: 400-800 mcg/day
- Vitamin C: 500-2,000 mg/day
- Vitamin E (as mixed tocopherols/tocotrienols): 200-400 IU/day
- Fish oil (omega-3 fatty acids): 2-4 g/day
- Vitamin D: 2,000-4,000 I.U./day

Chapter 4: The Not-So-Sweet Truth about Diabetes

Ask a dozen of your friends, co-workers and neighbors (or, if you're in an adventurous mood, take an informal poll among strangers on the street), and I bet that you'll find more than a few of them have diabetes. Like other chronic diseases I've talked about so far, diabetes, especially type-2 diabetes, wasn't very common back in our grandparents' day. Unfortunately, all that has changed.

Today, diabetes affects at least 35 million people in the United States, with the vast majority being type-2 diabetes. Obesity, which is fueling the spread of diabetes, is becoming more and more prevalent, so much so that it's been estimated that over 300 million people worldwide will have diabetes by 2025.

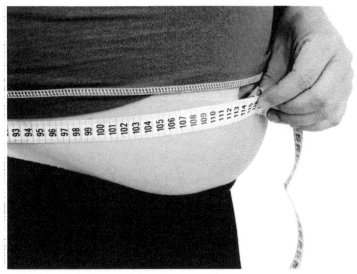

How fat are we?

Some statistics to mull over as you eat your triple-decker cheeseburger and drink your 64-ounce soda for lunch:

- Obesity in the United States increased by 61% between 1991 and 2000

- In 2015, experts estimated that 35of U.S. adults were obese

- 68% of American adults are overweight or obese (with a body mass index, or BMI, of over 25 kg/m)

What is BMI?

Read any newspaper or magazine article about obesity and you're sure to read about Body Mass Index, or BMI. BMI is calculated by dividing a person's weight in kilograms by the square of their height in meters. A normal BMI falls between 18.5 and 24.9; any higher than this and a person is considered either overweight (BMI between 25 and 29.9) or obese (BMI of 30 or greater).

Diabetes: the silent killer

So just what is diabetes? Simply put, diabetes is a condition in which the body does not produce or utilize insulin, a hormone secreted by the pancreas. Insulin is vital since it helps move glucose, or blood sugar, into every cell of your body. Your cells use glucose as fuel in much the same way your car uses gasoline. If your car runs out of gas, it stops running. If your cells can't get glucose—or if they can't utilize glucose—they don't work as well, if at all. And if your cells stop working, you stop working. Completely stop working. Which means—in no uncertain terms—you die.

What's the difference between type-1 and type-2 diabetes?

It's important to make the distinction between type-1 and type-2 diabetes (we'll leave type-3 diabetes to Chapter 1, since there still isn't a consensus whether it truly exists or not).

In type-1 diabetes, the pancreas doesn't produce enough, if any, insulin. In type-2 diabetes, your pancreas may not secrete enough insulin, or your cells may not be able to utilize insulin efficiently.

It's estimated that 10% of the 35 million Americans who have diabetes have type-1 diabetes, which is thought to be a genetic condition and usually starts very early in life. Type-2 diabetes, while having a genetic component, is largely thought to be a lifestyle disease—that is, a disease brought on by a sedentary way of life, obesity and a diet high in sugar and carbohydrates (in other words, the life that 90% of us Americans live).

The long-term consequences of untreated type-1 and -2 diabetes are the same, they include blindness, nerve damage, heart disease and premature death. And guys, remember that diabetes is one of the major causes of impotence. Now do I have your attention?

What are the differences between type-2 diabetes, insulin resistance and glucose intolerance?

You may have heard a friend mention that, while they don't have diabetes, their doctor told them to start monitoring their diet and exercising because they have insulin resistance or a glucose intolerance. But is there really a difference between these three conditions? Well, yes and no. Confused? That's okay—even doctors get confused about the difference. Let's take a minute to set it straight.

In simple terms, insulin resistance is the decreased ability of insulin to move glucose into cells. If you have insulin resistance, your pancreas, over time, will secrete more and more insulin in order to get glucose into the cells. However, sometimes getting more insulin isn't enough and glucose builds up in the blood. Other times the pancreas simply begins to "burn out" after so many years of overwork caused in part by a diet high in sugar from soft drinks, sweetened breakfast cereals, baked good and deserts. It's estimated that 50 million Americans are insulin resistant, and that figure is doing nothing but going up.

Glucose intolerance, otherwise known as impaired glucose tolerance (IGT), is diagnosed when your blood sugar level rises over a certain number after you drink a very sweet syrup. The test for IGT is done either at your doctor's office or a lab. If your pancreas is working like it should, even a big gulp of sugary-sweet syrup shouldn't cause your blood sugar to go up to a high level.

For all practical purposes, all people with type-2 diabetes are insulin resistant and have IGT, but not all people with insulin resistance or IGT have type-2 diabetes. However, without preventive measures and treatment, a huge percentage of patients with insulin resistance or IGT will go on to develop diabetes.

Diabetes: an epidemic among Hispanics

Anyone who knows me knows that I'm not into classifying people in any way, shape or form. To form an opinion—in non-politically correct terms, to judge someone—on how tall they are, what color their skin is or what sex they are is just plain stupid (and yes, I do realize that calling someone stupid probably is politically incorrect!). Yet there are times when it is important—at least medically—to know that your ethnicity and race do play a role. We do know that certain racial and ethnic groups suffer from certain diseases more than others; for example, children who develop cystic fibrosis are predomi-predominately from northern European heritage.

While diabetes is an equal opportunity killer, it does seem to strike some ethnic groups harder than others. It's estimated that over 1.5 million Hispanics have type-2 diabetes, and that number is rising every day. It's also known that type-2 diabetes is two to three times more common in Mexican-Americans and Puerto Ricans than it is in non-Hispanic Caucasians. The significant rise in obesity among Hispanic Americans is thought to be a significant factor in the incidence of diabetes among this group.

Diabetes: another multi-factorial disease

Like other chronic diseases, diabetes doesn't have just one cause. It's worth repeating that obesity, a sedentary lifestyle and a high-carb, high-sugar diet all take their toll and contribute to diabetes. Yet, as we learn more about diabetes, we also discover other underlying mechanisms that contribute to this condition.

Remember free radicals? (I'm sure you're saying, "Of course I remember—you talk about those damn things every chapter!") Well, they're back again, along with their old comrades, AGEs. Theoretically, the persistent levels of high blood sugars seen in pre-diabetic conditions, such as IGT and insulin resistance, cause a huge spike in the amount of AGEs produced throughout your body. AGEs then increase free radical production, which feeds AGE production, which causes even more free radical production, which leads to... well, you get the picture.

The diabetes belt is not a new fashion statement

In March of 2011, the CDC (Centers for Disease Control) designated an area consisting of 644 counties in 15 states (essentially the entire southeast quadrant of the United States) as a 'diabetes belt.'

"What does that mean?" some of you are probably asking. "Does it mean that if I live in North Carolina or Florida that there's something in the water that will give me diabetes?"

Fortunately, the answer to that question is no. What it means is that the CDC has identified a certain section of the U.S. that, for a variety of reasons, has a significantly higher number of people with type-2 diabetes than in other parts of the country. Reasons put forth by the CDC include the following:

Race—the south has a higher percentage of African-Americans (who are at higher risk of developing diabetes),

Obesity—the diabetes belt has a high percentage of people that are obese or morbidly obese,

Education and Socioeconomic status—the diabetes belt has a higher percentage of people without a college education and lower levels of income, both risk factors for developing type-2 diabetes.

So for you folks who live in the sunny south, don't despair: while you've been pigeonholed into yet another government-sponsored category, if you stay fit, eat well, and take my advice in the following pages, your chances of developing type-2 diabetes are no higher than your cousins living in the Midwestern rustbelt or other areas of this great country of ours.

Prescription medications for treating type-2 diabetes

If you're one of the tens of millions of people who have diabetes, you're probably overwhelmed at the number of diabetes medications out there. Some of the top-selling drugs in the U.S. (and the rest of the world) are for diabetes, including the following:

- <u>Sulfonylurea (glyburide, glimepiride, glipizide)</u>

  Sulfonylurea is the oldest oral medications used to control blood sugar. It works by prompting the pancreas to release more insulin. Sulfonylureas are often the first class of oral medications physicians use to control blood sugar levels in patients with type-2 diabetes.

- <u>Biguanide (metformin)</u>

  Biguanide works by slowing the release of glucose from the liver and increasing sensitivity of the muscles to insulin. It's often used in combination with sulfonylurea.

- <u>Thiazolidinediones (rosiglitazone, pioglitazone)</u>

  Like biguanide, thiazolidinediones help improve blood sugar levels by making cells in the body more sensitive to insulin. And like biguanide, thiazolidinediones are often used in combination with other drugs to treat type-2 diabetes.

- <u>Alpha-glucosidase inhibitors (acarbose, miglitol)</u>

  Alpha-glucosidase inhibitors can lower blood sugar levels (which often surge after meals) by blocking the digestive enzymes that break down carbohydrates.

Now, I hope you noticed that the heading for this section was for the treatment, not prevention, of diabetes. With the exception of acarbose (which I'll talk about more in a few pages), these medications treat, not prevent, diabetes. This is all fine and good, except that this book is about... let's hear everyone say it... prevention!

Type-2 diabetes is a preventable disease!

While it's been known for decades that insulin can significantly increase the lives of patients with type-1 diabetes, and prevent many secondary problems such as heart disease, kidney failure and blindness, the prevention of type-2 diabetes has proven to be harder to neatly isolate.

Aside from the reluctance of mainstream medicine to fully embrace prevention, one of the main reasons that type-2 diabetes is so prevalent is that it can take decades for any significant symptoms (blindness, heart attacks, impotence) to appear, but once they do appear, the damage has already been done.

If you have a family history of diabetes, or if you're overweight, love your high-carb foods (like potatoes, rice, pasta, bread, and corn) and never find time to exercise, make sure your doctor orders an annual fasting blood glucose test and hemoglobin A1C. Then, by incorporating lifestyle changes and taking safe, natural supplements, insulin resistance, glucose intolerance and type-2 diabetes will be three less things you will need to worry about later in life.

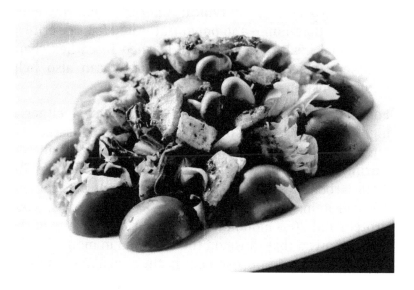

A healthy diet: key to avoiding type-2 diabetes

There should be no doubt that the typical Western diet (with its preponderance of sugars, starches and other carbohydrates) is a significant factor in the rise of type-2 diabetes over the last 30 years. Carbohydrates are broken down into glucose after being eaten, and this glucose is then shot right into your bloodstream. In contrast, fat, protein and fiber have very little immediate impact on blood sugar levels.

"But I watch what I eat," you might be saying to yourself. "I try to stay away from candy bars and cookies and only eat healthy food like whole grain bread." While I applaud your staying away from the junk food, you need to know that a piece of whole grain bread is still more than 80% starch. The bottom line is that a diet high in what I call the big bad 5—potatoes, rice, bread, corn (including corn syrup) and pasta—is fuel for the diabetes fire.

Besides our love of carbohydrates, it's my contention that both the government and major mainstream medical groups are to blame for the diabetes epidemic. By stigmatizing fats, these organizations have increased the amount of carbohydrates in the typical American diet. However, the fact is that mono- and polyunsaturated fats are critical to optimal health (as you have learned in earlier chapters) and, as research has shown, they can also help improve insulin resistance.

For instance, a study examined the effects of either a high-carbohydrate diet or a diet high in monounsaturated fat on insulin resistance in people with type-2 diabetes. During a 15-day period, the subjects ate either a diet with 40% carbohydrates, 40 percent monounsaturated fat and 20% protein, or a diet with 60% carbohydrates, 20% protein and 20% monounsaturated fat. The results of the study showed that those on the diet high in monounsaturated fat showed improvement in their insulin sensitivity compared to those subjects who ate a high-carbohydrate diet.

Now, I can already hear some of you saying, "Dr. Rosick, do you want me to eat nothing but raw vegetables and drink nothing but distilled water? I won't do it!" Guess what? I wouldn't do it either!

Have you heard of the Mediterranean diet? It was all the rage a few years ago, and for good reason: this diet, first described way back in the 1960s by Angel Keys and predominant in the (yes, you guessed it) Mediterranean region, is high in vegetables, fruits, nuts, legumes, lean meat and olive oil. In short, it is high in good fats and protein and low in simple carbs. Studies among men and women have shown that a Mediterranean diet can help lower blood glucose and serum insulin levels—in essence, it can lower your risk of diabetes. And you thought you couldn't eat well and avoid diabetes!

Using soy in the fight against diabetes

Increasing consumption of soy-based foods can have very healthy effects, especially for people who are prone to diabetes. Published studies have shown that, at least in post-menopausal women, incorporating soy into their diet can help prevent diabetes. In a randomized, crossover clinical trial, 42 post-menopausal women were assigned to a low-salt diet, a soy-protein diet (in which red meat was replaced with soy protein) or a soy-nut diet (in which red meat was replaced with soy nuts) for eight weeks. At the end of the study, the women eating the soy-nut diet had significantly decreased their insulin resistance and their fasting glucose levels. To me, this study is yet another example that simple dietary changes can literally change your health and your life.

Exercise: a key component in preventing diabetes

There is more to preventing diabetes than a diet low in carbohydrates, high in monounsaturated fats and full of vegetables, fruits, and fiber: many in the field of holistic health (including myself) think exercise is a key component of diabetes prevention. Multiple studies have shown exercise to improve insulin sensitivity and to consistently reduce insulin levels and fasting blood sugar levels.

"Yeah, yeah—you doctors push exercise for everything," you might be thinking. "I wanna see some proof!" Not a problem—in fact, there are three great studies showing the usefulness of exercise in preventing diabetes.

The first one is from China; there, over 100,000 men and women from all walks of life were screened for impaired glucose tolerance. Over a 6-year period, it was shown that those who exercised on a regular basis had a significantly decreased risk of developing type-2 diabetes.

The second study was from Finland; researchers looked at 522 middle-aged obese men and women over a three-year period. As in the Chinese study, those people who started and maintained an exercise regime while also increasing their vegetable and fiber intake had a relative reduction of 58% in the risk of developing diabetes.

The last study that I'll cite, which took place here in the good ol' U.S. of A., was dubbed the Diabetes Prevention Program (DPP). In this study, which cost over 170 million dollars, researchers looked at more than 3,800 men and women with IGT and randomly put them into three groups: one group received a placebo; another group received 850 grams of metformin twice daily; the third group received lifestyle intervention emphasizing a healthy diet and regular exercise. Over a follow-up time of approximately three years, the metformin group had a 31% decrease in the incidence of type-2 diabetes, while those in the lifestyle intervention group had a 58%

decrease in type-2 diabetes when compared to the placebo group.

These three studies show this fact, which should be shouted from the rooftops: you *can* prevent type-2 diabetes, even if you have insulin resistance or IGT, by incorporating a healthy low-carb, high-fiber, high-vegetable diet and regular exercise into your life. No need to pop a dozen pills a day or go to the doctor once a month for the rest of your life—diet and exercise alone can do it.

Another prescription medicine to prevent diabetes?

I'm certainly not one to just tell my patients to take another pill and see me next month. However, I'm not going to dismiss the good effects that metformin can have either. I am a realist, and I know that some people can't—or won't—significantly change their lifestyle or take supplements. Fortunately for these people, there are some prescription medications that may prevent diabetes.

Besides metformin, acarbose has also been shown in studies to reduce the incidence of type-2 diabetes. In the Study to Prevent Non-Insulin-Dependent Diabetes Mellitus (STOP-NIDDM), 1,368 people were randomly assigned to receive 100 milligrams of either a placebo or acarbose each day. Over a period of more than three years, researchers showed that the people taking acarbose had a 25% relative reduction in their risk of developing diabetes.

Can the amount of sleep you get influence your chances of developing diabetes?

Who among us gets enough sleep every night? I for one wouldn't raise my hand to that question. Unfortunately for me—and a great number of people who are sleep deprived—new research is coming forth showing that lack of sleep can increase your odds of developing diabetes.

In the *Journal of Clinical Endocrinology and Metabolism*, researchers presented evidence of a study on 11 healthy middle-aged men and women showing that those who decreased their nightly sleep time from 8.5 hours to 5.5 hours had changes in their blood sugar that was suggestive of an increased risk of diabetes. While larger studies are needed to confirm this preliminary data, this is just one more reason we all need to get a good night's sleep.

Natural supplements to prevent type-2 diabetes

Although I complained earlier about the government not doing nearly enough for prevention, I'm not going to complain about the Diabetes Prevention Program study. However, I do find it quite interesting how the government can spend over 170 million of our hard-earned tax dollars to study preventive medicine and not include any natural supplements.

"That's because supplements don't do any good," die-hard skeptics might say. "Why should the government waste money on expensive studies if supplements are just twenty-first century snake oil?" If this statement were true, I'd be in complete agreement; however, there are a number of safe, natural and inexpensive supplements that have been shown to help prevent type-2 diabetes.

Take magnesium, for instance. This simple mineral, which is often overlooked by the mainstream medical community (and by people who put together multi-million dollar studies like the DPP), has the potential to prevent type-2 diabetes.

"That's quite a statement, Dr. Rosick," you might be saying. "Can you back it up?" Of course, if you've read this far you already know the answer to that question!

In animal studies, supplemental magnesium has been shown to prevent the onset of diabetes in rats fed a high-sugar diet. Two well-documented human studies also show the vital role magnesium plays in preventing diabetes. In one study, researchers followed 85,060 women for 18 years and 42,872 men for 12 years. Their findings showed that men and women who had the highest consumption of magnesium also had the lowest rates of diabetes. Another study looked at 39,345 women for an average of 6 years; again, higher intakes of magnesium protected women against type-2 diabetes.

Studies like these make me wonder why magnesium doesn't get the respect it deserves when compared to prescription medications. Oh, that's right—magnesium doesn't have the push of a 170 million dollar government study.

Calcium and vitamin D: a one-two combination

Calcium and vitamin D, known for their combined ability to support bone health, may now have a new use—preventing diabetes. For three years in a double-blinded, randomized study, researchers followed 314 older men and women without diabetes and found that calcium and vitamin D supplements prevented further increases in blood glucose levels and protected against insulin resistance in people with impaired (elevated) fasting glucose levels.

In another study, researchers examined 126 healthy men and women and showed that higher blood levels of vitamin D corresponded with improved insulin sensitivity. The authors of the study concluded that people with low levels of vitamin D are at higher risk for insulin resistance.

Because these and other major studies, such as the Nurses Heath Study, show that vitamin D and calcium protect against diabetes, these two important supplements are certainly on my recommended list.

Chromium: mineral number two for diabetes prevention

Chromium picolinate is another mineral that has long been used to treat patients with type-2 diabetes and decreased insulin sensitivity. In an early study, researchers conducted a randomized, placebo-controlled study on 180 men and women with type-2 diabetes to see if chromium supplements could lead to metabolic improvements. Every day during the four-month study, the subjects either took 100 micrograms of chromium, 400 micrograms of chromium or a placebo. At the end of the study, there was a significant decrease in fasting glucose levels, fasting insulin levels, and two-hour insulin levels among the patients taking either the 100 or 400 mcg of chromium (but not in the placebo group),which points to an improvement in insulin resistance.

In another study, researchers gave middle-aged, obese men and women either a placebo or 1,000 micrograms of chromium daily. During the 8-month follow-up period, the researchers showed that people taking chromium had a significant increase in their insulin sensitivity.

While there hasn't yet been any large study on chromium's usefulness for directly preventing diabetes, I think the above studies—and others like them—give enough evidence for the use of this safe, inexpensive supplement in the prevention of type-2 diabetes.

Should middle-aged men take testosterone to prevent diabetes?

So far I've shown evidence that having optimal testosterone levels protects men against Alzheimer's, heart disease, and strokes. But that's just the start of the good news—testosterone also helps protect men against the ravages of diabetes.

A review article in *The Diabetes Educator* gave a succinct overview on the use of testosterone replacement therapy to prevent diabetes in aging men. Studies have consistently shown that testosterone levels are significantly lower in men with type-2 diabetes. Just as important, other studies have shown that men with higher testosterone levels had a 42% lower risk of developing type-2 diabetes! Now I don't know about you, but if a drug came out that could not only protect men against Alzheimer's, heart disease, and strokes—and could also decrease your chances of developing diabetes by 42%—men (and their significant others) would be breaking down their doctor's doors to get a prescription for it. Fortunately, that substance—testosterone—is already here, so make sure your doctor is routinely testing you for testosterone levels. If your level is low, and your doctor is willing -and knowledgeable—about testosterone replacement therapy, then start preventing diabetes now!

Cinnamon: not just for apple pie!

Cinnamon is a common, inexpensive spice used the world over. Now, laboratory and human studies are showing that this tasty spice may help prevent type-2 diabetes, thanks to a chemical component called methylhydroxychalcone polymer (MHCP).

Laboratory studies have shown that MHCP can improve cellular glucose metabolism, and human studies have shown that daily cinnamon consumption can significant improve insulin sensitivity. A randomized, placebo-controlled study published in *Diabetes Care* examined the effects of one, three, or six grams of cinnamon daily in 60 middle-aged men and women with type-2 diabetes. At the end of the 40-day study, the people taking cinnamon at any of the doses showed a significant decrease in their fasting serum glucose, triglycerides, total cholesterol, and LDL cholesterol. Now, I don't know about you, but if something as appetizing as cinnamon can lower blood sugar and cholesterol, I'm more than happy to find ways to incorporate it into my daily diet!

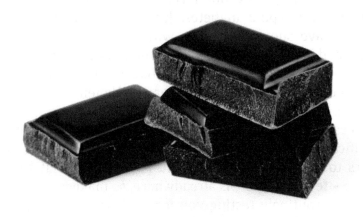

Chocolate: how something that tastes so good can be so good for you

I know that some sections of this book may seem a little depressing, so here's some news we can all be happy about: chocolate is good for you and may help prevent diabetes!

"Come on, Dr. Rosick, chocolate is good for you?" you may be saying to yourself. "Haven't you been saying that too much sugar is bad and can cause diabetes?" Well, yes, I have been saying that, but remember, chocolate, or more specifically, the cocoa that chocolate is made of, is an antioxidant-rich source of flavonoid polyphenols. Preliminary human studies have shown that dark chocolate (which is higher in polyphenols than white or milk chocolate) significantly improves insulin sensitivity. While more studies are certainly needed, I have no problem in telling my patients to choose a bar of dark organic chocolate if they need to indulge their sweet tooth now and then—it may actually protect them from diabetes.

A drink (or two) a day may keep diabetes away

So far, I've told you that a daily glass of red wine may protect you against Alzheimer's, heart disease, and strokes. Well guess what? Sipping a glass of wine at dinner or enjoying a beer while kicking back and watching football may help prevent diabetes. Studies show that having one to two drinks a day is associated with a 40% reduction in diabetes risk for men and a 60% to 70% risk reduction for women. One recent study—a 2-year, randomized, controlled trial done in Israel—showed that daily moderate wine consumption lead to an increase in HDL (the 'good' cholesterol) levels, a decrease in total cholesterol levels, and a decrease in fasting blood sugar levels. I don't necessarily recommend that non-drinkers run out and buy a case of beer or a couple gallons of wine, but if you enjoy your alcohol in moderation, feel free to go on enjoying it!

Antioxidants: their use just keeps growing and growing...

Let's see—so far I've told you that antioxidants are useful in preventing heart disease, Alzheimer's, cancer and strokes. Let's go ahead and add diabetes to the list.

Because oxidative damage contributes to diabetes, it makes perfect sense that antioxidants might help prevent diabetes, and recent studies have borne that line of thinking out. Studies have shown vitamin C to decrease fasting plasma insulin levels, and one long-term (23-year) study of thousands of middle-aged men and women found vitamin E to provide significant protection against the development of diabetes. Since vitamin C and vitamin E work together (vitamin C actually helps recycle vitamin

E so the body can use it again), I always tell my patients to use them together.

Lipoic acid: another antioxidant that can help prevent type-2 diabetes

I recommend lipoic acid to many of my patients; in particular, to my patients who are trying to prevent diabetes and to those who already suffer from it. In fact, lipoic acid is used in Germany to treat diabetic polyneuropathies—that is, damage to the nerves caused by diabetes. I've also used it for patients suffering from this painful and debilitating consequence of diabetes, and I have seen amazing results.

Studies have shown that as little as 600 milligrams a day of lipoic acid can significantly improve insulin sensitivity. We don't know exactly how lipoic acid does this, but we do know that that lipoic acid helps maintain levels of glutathione (see chapters 1 and 3), which may help decrease oxidative damage that contributes to and is brought about by type-2 diabetes.

Fighting diabetes with an old lunch favorite

How many of use went to school as kids with a peanut butter sandwich packed in our lunchboxes courtesy of mom? Turns out that mom may have been giving us more than a tasty snack—she may have been protecting us from diabetes.

Researchers have been combing over the data from the Nurses' Health Study, a humongous project that collected data from over 83 thousand nurses. One of the many conclusions they came up with was that women who ate peanut butter 5 or more times a week—compared with those who never/almost never ate peanut butter—had a significantly decreased risk of developing diabetes. Yet just another example of proving how moms almost always do what's best for us, whether they know it or not!

A morning cup of coffee may help prevent diabetes

In chapter 1, I said that coffee might protect against Alzheimer's. In chapter 3 I said that coffee might lessen the risk of strokes. Now it turns out that coffee may also protect you against diabetes. A study published in 2006 showed that consumption of coffee (both caffeinated and decaf) among women aged 26 to 46 was inversely related to the development of type-2 diabetes. Another study that followed 910 men and women aged 50 and greater, showed that coffee consumption helped protect against the development of diabetes, even in people with impaired glucose tolerance. Finally, a more recent study examined the effects of coffee in 6,974 men and 7,655 women aged 35 to 64 and found that coffee consumption seemed to protect against type-2 diabetes. Although the researchers conducting these studies can't say just why coffee is protective, why not drink coffee in the morning both to get your motor running and to help protect against type-2 diabetes?

The bottom line: prevent diabetes now or pay dearly later

The epidemic of diabetes is especially galling to me and to other physicians trained in preventive medicine. Type-2 diabetes is one chronic disease that even some of those in mainstream medicine acknowledge (though not loudly enough, in my opinion) can be prevented. If you want to spare yourself decades of expensive prescription drugs and an increased risk of blindness, strokes, heart attack and—for men—impotence, please discuss with your doctor the following methods you can incorporate into your life right now to prevent diabetes!

Strategies to prevent diabetes

<u>Behavioral Tips</u>

- Exercise 20 to 30 minutes, three to four times a week

- Eat a diet high in vegetables, fiber, protein and nuts; low in foods with simple carbs and starches (such as potatoes, rice, bread and pasta)

- Enjoy your morning cup of coffee and your evening glass of wine—no need to feel guilty!

- Get at least 8 to 9 hours of sleep at night

<u>Supplements</u>

- Magnesium: 400-800 mg/day

- Vitamin D: 1,000-2,000 IU/day

- Chromium: 100-400 mcg/day

- Vitamin E (as mixed tocopherols/tocotrienols): 200-400 IU/day

- Vitamin C: 500-2,000 mg/day

- Alpha lipoic acid: 200-600 mg/day

Chapter 5: The Never-Ending War on Cancer

With the eradication of formerly deadly diseases such as smallpox and polio, it's no longer unusual for people to live well into their 70s, 80s and even 90s. Yet, despite all of our scientific prowess, there is an area in which the medical community is making no headway, regardless of the decades of research and billions of taxpayer dollars. That is the war on cancer.

In 1971, President Nixon declared war on cancer and directed the economic and scientific might of the federal government against this deadly disease. Since that time, the United States government (funded by us, the taxpayers) has spent approximately 50 billion dollars to find a cure for cancer. Yet today that cure appears as distant as it did all those years ago. It's estimated that this year alone, approximately 1.4 million Americans will be diagnosed with cancer and close to 600,000 will die from it. A report in the widely respected journal *Oncologist* stated that in cancer will strike 1 in 2 men and 1 in 3 women in the United States.

"But Dr. Rosick, I just heard on the news last night that we're winning the war on cancer and that more people than ever are being cured!" If you are thinking that, you would be right—lately, there has been a lot of good news about cancer from the American Cancer Society (ACS) and the National Cancer Institute (NCI). But it's wise to remember that medical statistics can be spun just as well as a political campaign message.

The sad fact is that five-year survival rates for all cancers have remained virtually static since 1971. The incidence of cancers not predominately caused by smoking, such as non-Hodgkin's lymphoma, multiple myeloma and adult brain cancer, are increasing at alarming rates. Despite billions of dollars in research and expensive new pharmaceuticals, the cancer epidemic continues to affect almost everyone. Every day, I see that pain reflected in the eyes of my patients whom I have to tell that horrible news no doctor wants to give: "you have cancer."

Cancer has hit me on a very personal level. It has taken the life of my grandfather, my aunt, my mother-in-law, my great uncle and a number of cousins. In 1992, during my third year of medical school, metastatic esophageal cancer took the life of my father. For nine months, I watched him turn from a strong, vigorous man into an 80-pound skeleton of skin and bones, all while receiving hundreds of thousands of dollars' worth of chemotherapy and radiation, which did absolutely nothing except worsen his misery and speed up his death. Finally, in May of 2010, my mother was diagnosed with leukemia, the same type (AML) that had taken her sister 15 years earlier. For 2 months, my mother was treated with the widely accepted mainstream medicine regime of hospitalization and chemotherapy, only to suffer the same heart-wrenching results that my father did: on July 27, 2010, two short months after diagnosis, she died. As a sobering postscript, the very expensive—and FDA approved—chemo my mother was getting for her cancer, Mylotarg, was suddenly pulled off the market just after she had received her last dose. It seems that the FDA looked over data regarding the drug, which made unknown millions of dollars for its manufacturer and the oncologists who ordered it. Not only did Mylotarg NOT work in treating AML, it actually increased patients' chances of dying. Unfortunately, it only took the FDA 10 years (Mylotarg was given the FDA holy stamp of approval in 2000) to figure this out.

So if I seem more impassioned, more opinionated and more angry about the way mainstream medicine has both widely and blindly embraced the costly (and often deadly) twin sisters of chemo and radiation while snubbing and belittling preventive & integrative measures and more innovative (and less expensive) approaches to cancer treatment... it's because I am.

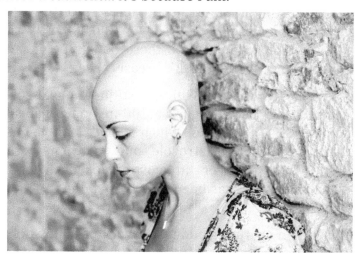

Prevention: the key to stopping the cancer epidemic

According to many in mainstream medicine, the solution to the cancer epidemic is to continue pouring money into cancer diagnosis and treatment. Both the National Cancer Institute (with a yearly budget of about five billion dollars) and the American Cancer Society (with a yearly budget of about one billion dollars) spend the vast majority of their money on diagnosis and treatment, and not on prevention. However, a small, but growing group of leading cancer researchers, like Dr. Samuel S. Epstein (head of the National Cancer Prevention Coalition and author of numerous books and articles on the causes of cancer) are calling for a major overhaul in the way that the federal government spends our tax dollars to fight cancer. These researchers recommend focusing on preventive measures to stop the disease in the first place— what a concept!

Prevention loses at the National Cancer Institute

Breast cancer. These two words strike fear in the heart of women everywhere, and for good reason—breast cancer is the most common cancer in women, Breast cancer rates in the United States have tripled since the 1960s; this year alone, there will be over 200,000 new cases diagnosed. You'd think that if there's one type of cancer that needs to be prevented, it's breast cancer.

For a while, the National Cancer Institute thought so, too. In fact, the NCI had designed a 100-million-dollar study called the STELLAR trial, which would look to see if certain medications (letrozole and raloxifene) could prevent breast cancer in post-menopausal women. Unfortunately, trial has been put on hold due to "budgetary constraints."

Let's see—an operating budget of over five billion dollars, hundreds of thousands of new cases of breast cancer a year, and the NCI can't find the money for a preventive study? Never mind not funding studies using natural supplements to prevent cancer—how can people justify stopping a study to prevent breast cancer?

What causes cancer, and how do we stop it?

Dr. Epstein and other advocates of cancer prevention point out that the development of cancer is not a one-step process—rather, cancer is a multi-stage disease that in its earliest stages is quite responsive to prevention. Yet, before we talk about how to prevent cancer, let's take a few minutes to look at what cancer is and what causes it.

Cancer occurs when cells in your body duplicate out of control. Normally, the cells in your body divide over and over again at a certain rate and then die (a process called apoptosis) before being replaced by new, younger cells. Cancerous cells divide faster and faster, crowding out and eventually killing non-cancerous cells; they also spread throughout the body, a process called metastasis. Metastasis is one of the things that make curing cancer so damn hard. While a surgeon may be able to cut out a cancerous tumor in your colon, cells from that tumor may have already spread throughout your body, not to show up as full-blown cancer for years.

Now we know what the enemy is; next, we need to know how the enemy forms. That's a question we'd all like answered, and while we have some clues, the final report isn't in just yet. What we do know is that there are multiple factors that cause cancer, with two of the most prominent being heredity and behavior.

Heredity

We know that some cancers, such as breast cancer, retinoblastoma, and Wilms' tumors, are inherited. Additionally, some people are more genetically prone to cancer than others. We've all heard the story of a 95 year-old grandma who smoked two packs of unfiltered cigarettes a day and never got cancer. Fortunately for this grandma, she had some (as yet) unknown genetic resistance to cancer. However, even if this were your grandma, I wouldn't advise betting your health—or your life—on having those same genes.

Behavior

Unlike your genetic makeup, you can change your behavior to give yourself the best possible chance of avoiding cancer. First off is smoking. In Chapter 2, I explained how smoking causes heart disease and told you how to get off cigarettes, so I won't go over any of that again. However, I will tell you that at least 30% of all cancer deaths (that's right, all cancers, not just lung cancer) in the U.S. are attributed to smoking. Smoking is thought to cause at least 17 types of cancer, including the following:

- Colon cancer
- Esophageal cancer
- Kidney cancer
- Laryngeal cancer
- Liver cancer
- Lung cancer
- Myeloid leukemia
- Nasal cavity and paranasal sinus cancer
- Oral cancer
- Pancreatic cancer
- Pharyngeal cancer
- Rectal cancer
- Stomach cancer
- Bladder cancer
- Uterine and cervical cancer

Need I say more about smoking and cancer?

Two other common and cancer-promoting behaviors are alcohol consumption and unprotected sex. Now, I can already hear the protests: "Come on, Doc, we'll quit smoking, but don't ask us to give up booze and sex!" Hear me out. I told you in earlier chapters that reducing stress (through activities like sex) and consuming alcohol in moderation were healthy things to do, and I'm not about to tell you otherwise. However, you need to know that studies have associated high levels of alcohol consumption (defined as at least 3 to 4 drinks a day) with higher rates of certain cancers.

It's also known that having unprotected sex (that is, sex without a condom) can lead to the transmission of human papillomaviruses, or HPVs, which can cause cervical and anal cancer. If you engage in unprotected sex with a partner whose sexual history is a mystery to you, you put yourself at risk for an HPV infection (as well as all sorts of other nasty diseases), which can lead to certain forms of cancer.

The connection between stress and cancer

Have I stressed you out by talking about sex and alcohol? I hope not, since many people now think that stress—especially if it isn't dealt with in a timely fashion—can lead to many of the chronic diseases I've talked about, including cancer.

"Come on, Dr. Rosick, stress is all in your mind—how can that cause cancer?" you might be asking. It's a good question, and I have a good answer. The mind influences the body (and vice-versa) through the (take a deep breath here) hypothalamic-pituitary-adrenal (HPA) axis. This intricate connection between the brain and the endocrine system exerts a wide influence over our health, and many researchers suggest that our stressful twenty-first-century lifestyles are overtaxing the HPA axis, leading to diseases such as cancer.

Before we discuss how aberrations of the HPA axis contribute to chronic disease, let's take a few minutes to go over the basics of how the HPA axis works. It starts in the brain with the hypothalamus, a specialized gland in the brain that some consider the master gland of the neuro-endocrine system.

The hypothalamus has many functions, such as controlling body temperature, water balance, thirst and hunger. It also controls the pituitary gland, a small, bean-sized structure that sits just below the hypothalamus. During times of stress, the hypothalamus releases corticotropin-releasing factor (CRF), which signals the pituitary gland to release adrenocorticotropic hormone (ACTH). This hormone then travels through the bloodstream to the adrenals, two small, triangle-shaped glands located on the top of the kidneys. When ACTH reaches the adrenals, it causes them to release a biochemical known as cortisol.

Cortisol: the stress hormone

Cortisol is, in many ways, a paradoxical hormone. You need a certain amount of cortisol to maintain optimal health, but if there's too much or too little, the results can be deadly. Cortisol is involved in a number of bodily functions, including blood pressure regulation, cardiovascular and immunological functioning, and the metabolism of fats, proteins and carbohydrates. In stressful situations, cortisol is secreted at higher-than-normal rates to help the body break down and utilize fatty acids and proteins for energy production, which is especially important for optimal brain functioning. Unlike hormones such as testosterone and DHEA, cortisol levels generally don't decrease as you get older.

How stress can kill

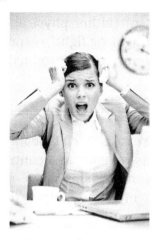

While those of us well versed in integrative medicine take the relationship between the mind and body very seriously, it's only recently come about that mainstream medicine has paid any attention to the ways emotions and stress can affect our body. That's surprising, because it's been known since Hans Selye's landmark work in 1936 that, because of the interaction between the mind and the adrenal glands, both psychological and biological stress can negatively affect health.

In 1946, Selye published his now-classic work on the link between chronic stress and disease. Through careful observation, Selye reasoned that living organisms, including humans, react to both physical and psychological stressors in a predictable physiological pattern that maintain homeostasis—a constant, dynamic metabolic equilibrium in which all organ systems function in order to maintain optimal health. He termed these often-complex physiological and behavioral responses to stress the General Adaptation Syndrome. Selye also observed that when stress was continuous, the organism would ultimately burn out and die. This observation led Selye to devise the following three-step model to describe the General Adaptation Syndrome:

Step 1: Alarm Reaction

An immediate stressor (either physical or psychological) activates both the "flight or fight" response and the HPA axis, leading to an increased production of hormones such as cortisol.

Step 2: Resistance Phase

If the perceived stressors aren't dealt with in a timely fashion, the HPA axis remains in a continual 'on' mode in order to maintain homeostasis; as a result, adrenal hypertrophy and a myriad of other deleterious health effects begin to occur.

Step 3: Exhaustion Phase

When stress is prolonged, the adrenal glands, as well as other organ systems, begin to burn out and their function declines precipitously. If the exhaustion phase continues long enough, the organism will die.

Chronic stress and increased cortisol levels can contribute to multiple illnesses

It's been 90+ years since Hans Selye's landmark work on the relationship between stress, high cortisol levels and illness was published. Since then, a number of studies have confirmed many of Selye's observations. Both acute and chronic stress have been shown to contribute to abnormally high levels of cortisol.

The dangerous connection between chronic stress, cortisol and cancer

Since the late 1990s, scientists have presented provocative evidence linking cancer, stress and elevated cortisol levels. A 1996 paper in the journal *Psychoneuroendocrinology*, examined HPA hormonal levels in women with both early-stage and metastatic breast cancer. In this case-control study, researchers showed that women with both types of breast cancer had higher levels of cortisol than women without breast cancer. A more recent report in the journal *Lancet Oncology* summarized what is currently known about the complex interactions between the HPA system, stress and cancer. The authors stated that stress taxes your immune system, which may hinder the immune system from protecting you against a variety of illnesses—including cancer.

Night-shift workers may be at greater risk for cancer

In my younger days—when there were no gray hairs on my head—I would occasionally work the midnight shift, and I detested it. Even though I'd sleep (somewhat) during the day, I never felt like myself. Now, research is showing that working the night shift may do more than just make you feel crummy—it may predispose you to cancer. It's thought, but not yet proven, that this may be due to the suppression of melatonin, a hormone that experimental studies have shown to have anti-cancer activity.

Normally, melatonin levels are high at night, when it's dark, and low during the day, when it's light. However, artificial lighting suppresses melatonin level in night-shift workers. Studies on nurses working night shifts have shown that women who work rotating night shifts at least three nights per month have an increased risk of breast and colorectal cancer.

Free radicals and AGEs

You didn't think I was going to skip over free radicals and AGEs in this chapter, did you? As I've shown you, these dastardly cousins are involved in most chronic diseases, and that doesn't exclude cancer.

Multiple scientific papers have provided evidence that AGEs contribute to cancer. One early paper from the 1990s detailed the role of AGEs in the development of pancreatic cancer. A more recent article, published in the journal *Investigative Dermatology*, examined the involvement of AGEs in the growth and metastasis of melanoma, the deadliest type of skin cancer. The authors came to the conclusion that "AGE[s] might be involved in the growth and invasion of melanoma..."

Of course, free radicals are just as bad. Numerous studies have shown that free-radical damage to your cells, and in particular, to the DNA in your cells, may be a significant cause of cancer. Fortunately, studies also show that compounds such as vitamin C, vitamin E, selenium, carotenoids, glutathione and phytochemicals are all potent antioxidants that can stop the damaging effects of free radicals, potentially protecting us against cancer.

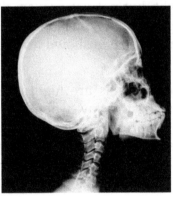

Do medical X-rays cause cancer?

My patients often come to me with various complaints, from shoulder injuries to abdominal pain, and expect to have an X-ray. It seems that for many people, getting an X-ray done at their physician's office is just part of a normal exam. Of course, I certainly don't hesitate to order an X-ray when it is warranted; however, I also explain to my patients that an X-ray is not a benign procedure.

It's now quite clear that X-rays can exert a dangerous effect on the human body. X-rays are a form of ionizing radiation, a type of electro-magnetic radiation that physicists refer to as high energy. Each X-ray particle can penetrate most solid substances, including the human body. In contrast, visible light, which is another form of radiation, is much less energetic and can be stopped by something as simple as paper or cloth.

When ionizing radiation enters the body, it transfers some of its energy to cells in the body as it passes through. This transfer of energy can cause complex, irreparable damage to the cell and its DNA. If the damage is great enough, the cell will die. However, if the cell doesn't die, the genetic damage caused by the ionizing radiation can induce both benign and malignant (cancerous) tumors.

The damage caused by X-rays accumulates throughout a person's life, with each dose of ionizing radiation causing more and more damage. It doesn't matter to your cells if an X-ray was given 20 years ago or 20 minutes ago—the cellular and genetic damage is the same. And enough damage can cause cancer.

A multitude of scientific studies show that exposure to X-rays, especially early in life, may be a cause of a number of cancers, including the following:

- Bladder cancer
- Brain cancer
- Breast cancer
- Central nervous system cancer
- Colon cancer
- Leukemia
- Lung cancer

- Ovarian cancer

- Salivary gland cancer

- Skin cancer

- Stomach cancer

- Thyroid cancer

Dr. John W. Gofman believes that medical X-rays are a significant cause of the cancer and heart disease epidemics in America. In an exhaustively researched 699-page book called *Radiation and Human Health*, Dr. Gofman presents data, based on mortality rates among 130 to 250 million people, to support his hypothesis that "over 50 percent of the death rate from cancer today, and over 60 percent of the death rate from ischemic heart disease today, are X-ray induced."

Dr. Gofman's book should be read by all physicians, and by all patients, too. Yet although he presents chapter after chapter of meticulous studies to prove his hypothesis, Dr. Gofman is by no means against the use of X-rays for clearly defined medical studies. What Dr. Gofman does make clear is that physicians should use X-rays and other forms of ionizing radiation as carefully as they use other mediations.

Gofman's claims were recently bolstered by a study in the respected British medical journal *The Lancet* linking medical X-rays to cancer in Europe and the United States. According to the authors, the growing use of CT (Computerized Tomography) scans, a popular way of imaging body organs, is responsible for the largest number of cancer cases, followed by barium enemas (X-rays of the large intestine), hip X-rays and pelvis X-rays. In no uncertain terms, the authors conclude that there is no safe threshold dose for ionizing radiation (X-rays).

"Are you telling us we should never get X-rays?" you might be asking. No. X-rays, CT scans and other uses of ionizing radiation are very important tools in a physician's bag of tricks and I'll continue to use them judiciously. But, I will always keep in mind—and educate my patients on—their possible side effects.

Our chemical—and cancerous—modern society

Since World War II, tens of thousands of new chemicals have been introduced into our environment (and if they're in the environment, eventually they'll end up in you and me). While many of these chemicals have allowed us to enjoy prosperity and comfort, we should remember, as my father used to tell me, that everything has a price. And the price of these man-made chemicals may be an epidemic of cancer.

In his meticulously researched book, *Cancer-Gate* (which I urge all of you to read), Dr. Epstein details how drowning our environment—and ourselves—in a toxic soup of chemicals, has fed the growing cancer epidemic. Particularly eye opening is Dr. Epstein's list of what he called the "dirty dozen consumer products," everyday household goods that actually contain cancer-causing substances. Included in the list are following:

- Garden and lawn weed killers with the herbicide 2,4-D
- Hair coloring products with quaternium-15 and phenylene-diamines
- Household cleaners with crystalline silica
- Household spray cleaners with orthophenylphenol
- Makeup with BHA
- Dog and cat flea collars with propoxur
- Toothpaste with FD and C Blue #1 coloring

Pesticide exposure linked to brain cancer

Walk into the gardening section of any large store like Wal-Mart and you'll see row after row of pesticides. While you might think, "They must be safe or the government wouldn't allow them to be sold," think again—a report published in the journal *Occupational and Environmental Medicine* shows that pesticide exposure may increase your risk of brain cancer, yet despite this information, pesticides are still sold in abundance at most local gardening stores.

In a study of almost 700 adults with brain tumors in France, researchers found that in agricultural workers—who have a high exposure to commonly used pesticides—risk of developing brain cancer was 29% greater than it was in people without exposure to pesticides. Even more frightening, the researchers found that people who used pesticides around their house were twice as likely to be diagnosed with brain cancer than people who didn't use household pesticides.

Diabetes isn't the only disease to have a belt

Remember the last chapter, when I talked about the diabetes belt? Cancer also has a belt—of sorts—that's been clearly defined in a report by the National Resources Defense Council. Entitled "Health Alert: Disease Clusters Spotlight the Need to Protect People from Toxic Chemicals," this report—which I urge you to download and read—highlights different areas of the country that have unusually high incidences of cancer and other deadly diseases. From California to my own home state of Michigan, this Health Alert highlights the continuing danger of toxic chemicals and where these "cancer belts" are. Again, like I said to the people in the diabetes belt, don't feel that you have to drop all your belongings and move if you happen to live near—or in—one of these toxic zones. Use the information to take smart preventive measures, and maybe even write your congressmen and women so that they use some of our tax dollars to do more than just go on junkets to Europe; how about using it to clean up our environment and decrease our risk of dying from cancer and other deadly diseases?

Prevention is the best protection against cancer

While curing cancer is still just a dream for hundreds of thousands of people, you can start NOW to prevent cancer from occurring in the first place. While it would take a whole new book (which I plan to write in the not-too-distant future) to list all the ways in which one can prevent cancer from occurring (as well as re-occurring for those who've been previously diagnosed with it), below is a practical list that you and your loved ones can start now so you can avoid becoming another heart-breaking statistic in the "war on cancer."

I. Behavioral Changes

1. Quit smoking. Do I really need to beat you over the head about this? I didn't think so. If you need some tips on how to do this, feel free to skip back to Chapter 2.

2. Drink in moderation. How do I define moderation? Easy—no more than 2 drinks a day. Now I'm not saying that if you're spending a summer afternoon at a friend's house (and NOT driving home) you can't have more than that—I'm just saying that any more than 2 or so drinks a day can put you at an increased risk of developing cancer.

3. Avoid risky sex. Again, like quitting smoking, this should pretty much be a no-brainer.

4. Monitor your medical X-ray exposure. One of the big things now in some forms of preventive medicine is a "whole body CT scan." While CT scans can be lifesaving, a whole body CT scan, just for the sake doing one, is not only expensive, but will give you significant exposure to

ionizing radiation. If your doctor orders an X-ray, CT scan, or bone scan, and you're not sure why, ask her or him. If she or he can't give you a good reason for it, then find yourself another doctor!

5. Learn to read labels on food and household goods. Learn to be a smart and cancer-conscious shopper, and only buy those foods and household goods that aren't full of cancer-causing chemicals (for a detailed listing of these, look up Dr. Epstein's book or go to the Environmental Working Group's website at www.ewg.org that lists the health-safety of over 15,000 name-brand products).

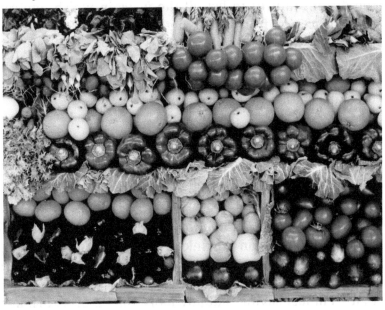

II. Diet & Supplements

One of the most widely available methods of cancer prevention, yet essentially overlooked at best (and ridiculed at worst) by major cancer organizations and mainstream medicine, is the use of natural chemopreventive agents. Over 250 case-control and cohort studies have been done on natural chemopreventive agents such as those found in fruits and vegetables, and the data is overwhelming and non-refutable—there is a significant inverse relationship between the consumption of fruits and vegetables and the incidence of cancer.

A number of phytochemical and other compounds that I've already discussed in earlier chapters can help prevent cancer, and what follows are what I like to call (take a deep breath): "Dr. Rosick's ABCs of cancer-preventing phytochemicals and the foods that contain them."

1. Allyl Sulfides—found in garlic (more on these below) and onions, these biochemicals stop the growth of cancerous cells and cause apotosis in pre-cancerous cells.

2. Anthocyanins—found in grapes, black currants, & mangosteen, these substances are powerful antioxidants and help prevent metastasis.

3. Carotenoids—found in carrots, pumpkins, and winter squash, one of these cancer-fighting compounds, beta-carotene (which some of you are probably familiar with) got some very bad press a few years ago. Seems that smokers who took beta-carotene increased their risk of cancer. However, don't let this one study dissuade you from carotenoids, since a number of studies have shown that an overall higher intake of carotenoids decreases your risk for a number of cancers.

4. Catechins—found in green tea, catechins are more powerful antioxidants.

5. Ellagic acid—found in fruits such as raspberries, strawberries, and grapes, this substance has been shown in animal studies to protect against colon and esophageal cancer.

6. Isoflavones—found in soy. These are so important I've expanded on them in the following section.

7. Lutein—found in mangos and squash, this powerful antioxidant is also useful in protecting against macular

degeneration, one of the leading causes of blindness in the elderly.

8. Lycopene—found in tomatoes and watermelon, lycopene has been shown in numerous studies to provide protection against the development of prostate cancer.

9. Quercetin—found in most fruits and vegetables, quercetin acts as a powerful antioxidant.

10. Resveratrol—found in grapes, this powerful antioxidant is useful not only for cancer prevention but also for prevention of heart disease and strokes.

11. Sulforaphane—found in cruciferous vegetables such as broccoli, cauliflower, and Brussels sprouts, this vitally important chemical promotes apoptosis and detoxifies potential carcinogens.

Nutritional approaches to preventing cancer

1. Garlic: a malodorous cancer fighter

It seems that there's no middle ground when it comes to garlic—people either love it or hate it. I love it; for me, just about any food tastes better with garlic. While this makes it important that I bring mouthwash and a toothbrush when I eat out, it may also help protect me against cancer. Numerous studies have shown that a high intake of garlic may protect you against the following cancers:

- Stomach cancer
- Colon cancer
- Rectal cancer
- Breast cancer
- Prostate cancer
- Laryngeal cancer

With a list like that, maybe it's time that those of you who don't enjoy the pungent aroma and taste of garlic to think about changing your tastes!

2. Spice up your foods

If you don't like the taste of garlic, how about spicing up your food with ginger and turmeric? These spices, which belong to the Zingiberaceae family, contain potent anti-cancer agents.

Ginger and turmeric have been used for centuries in traditional Asian medicine, and modern science is finally catching up with the wisdom of our elders. Population-based studies have shown that people in Southeast Asian countries—where ginger and turmeric are as common as salt and pepper in America—have significantly lower rates of colon cancer, gastrointestinal cancer, prostate cancer and breast cancer. Multiple laboratory and animal studies have shown that ginger possesses a multitude of anti-cancer properties. Turmeric has also been shown to help prevent cancer. A review article in the journal *Food and Chemical Toxicology* listed a number of ways in which turmeric promotes its cancer-fighting abilities including fighting inflammation and free radicals.

"But what about human studies?" I can hear the cynics cry. "There have been no long-term human studies showing that turmeric and ginger can really prevent cancer!" That's true. There have been no government-sanctioned studies on these spices conducted by researchers who are biased against natural agents to prevent cancer. And to that I say...so what?

Millions of people consume large amounts of turmeric and ginger daily with no ill effects; as a population, these people show significantly decreased rates of cancer when compared to Western populations that don't use these spices. If we wait for a definitive study, millions of us will have already lost in the war against cancer. If you want to wait for this study, be my guest. In the meantime, I'll continue to encourage my patients to spice their foods with ginger and turmeric.

3. Soy: an important chemopreventive agent

If there's one gift from God with great potential for preventing cancer, it's soy. This tiny bean has been extensively studied and is touted by some in the holistic medical field as the answer to all cancers. While I think that's an overstatement, I have read enough to know that adding soy-based foods to your diet might very well protect you against cancer later in life.

Many researchers think that soy gets its cancer-fighting ability from phytochemical constituents called isoflavones. Two of the most well-known isoflavones are genistein and daidzein. Many integrative medical practitioners, and a small, but growing number of mainstream practitioners, now believe that consumption of soy and isoflavones can significantly reduce the risk of many chronic diseases, including cancer, heart disease and diabetes.

Soy and breast cancer

Significant interest in soy and isoflavones as anti-cancer agents began in the 1990s when studies showed that Asian women, who consume approximately 700 times the amount of isoflavones than American women, have significantly lower risks of developing breast cancer. Because animal studies indicate that both a diet high in soy and genistein can protect against breast cancer, colon cancer and skin tumors, it seems reasonable to think that soy can help prevent human cancers; in particular, breast cancer.

In a population-based prospective study of 21,852 Japanese women aged 40 to 59, researchers found that women with high intakes of soy isoflavones were protected against breast cancer.

Soy can also protect men

While it's exciting to know that soy-based products can help protect women from breast and endometrial cancer, it's also comforting to know that soy isoflavones can also help protect men from prostate cancer, the second leading cancer killer of men. Every year, prostate cancer affects about 230,000 men and kills approximately 30,000. Large epidemiological studies have shown that men in Asia, who consume large amounts of soy-based foods, have a significantly lower incidence of prostate cancer than their Western counterparts.

One of the largest human studies conducted here in the U.S. was a prospective study on 12,395 men in Loma Linda, California, between 1976 and 1992. During that time period, researchers showed that men who drank more than one glass of soy milk a day showed a 70% reduction in the risk of prostate cancer when compared to men who did not drink soy milk.

Soy and skin cancer

As if protection against breast cancer and prostate cancer weren't enough, new studies show that genistein may provide protection against skin aging caused by sun exposure and may even inhibit skin cancer. In a report in the *Journal of Nutrition*, researchers at the Mount Sinai School of Medicine examined the effects of both oral and topical genistein on ultraviolet (UV) radiation-induced skin cancer in mice. In mice that either drank water fortified with genistein or had genistein directly applied to their skin, there was a significant decrease in cancer formation. The researchers also showed that when applied directly to human skin, genistein substantially decreased photo damage from UV radiation.

Yogurt may keep cancer away

When I was a child, my mom "suggested" that I eat yogurt. "It's good for you!" I remember her saying just as clearly as I remember turning my nose up and pushing the yogurt away. Now, years older and a bit wiser, I eat yogurt at least once a day, both because I like the taste and because of the many healthful benefits.

"I've heard yogurt is full of bacteria," you might be thinking. "Isn't it dumb to eat something full of bacteria?" Well, no—the bacteria in yogurt are actually good for you. The good bacteria (probiotics) in yogurt do many useful things: they produce natural antibiotics to keep bad bacteria out of your digestive tract, they help with digestion, they produce B-vitamins in your small intestine and they strengthen your immune system.

In addition, probiotics may also protect us from certain forms of cancer. By strengthening your immune system, probiotics may help fight off cancer in its earliest stages. Probiotics also increase acidity in the colon, which may protect against colon cancer. Finally, probiotics may prevent cancer by reducing levels of pro-cancerous enzymes in the gut.

As you might have guessed, there have been no large, federally funded studies on probiotics and their effect on cancer. But so what? You can wait for the Feds to get off their bureaucratic butts and do the right thing, or you can take charge of your own health. Eating yogurt once or twice a day or taking a probiotic supplement can keep your digestive tract happy and may protect you against cancer, so what are you waiting for?

Are supplements enough?

Many of my patients don't really like eating fruits and vegetables. Sometimes they ask if they can just take supplements to protect themselves against cancer. While many of my mainstream medical colleagues would answer with an emphatic no, I'll be a bit gentler and kinder. While study after study has shown that phytochemicals and vitamins in fruits and vegetables can protect you from cancer, not as many studies have shown that supplements provide the same benefits. However, there still is enough evidence for me to recommend the following supplements, especially to people whose still consume the standard American diet (SAD) of fast food, processed food, and soda multiple days a week.

B-vitamins

The B vitamins (B1, B2, B6, B12 and folate) are water-soluble vitamins (meaning that you don't store them in your body) that are on my base recommendation list for new patients asking which supplements they should take. Aside from being essential to proper brain and nerve function, B-vitamins may protect you against cancer.

Two studies published in the *Journal of the National Cancer Institute* (certainly not a bastion of alternative medicine!) showed that increased levels of folate and vitamin B6 might protect women against breast cancer and ovarian cancer. In another study, published in the *Journal of Clinical Nutrition*, researchers looked at over 11,000 women and their risk of invasive breast cancer. The researchers reported that women who had the highest folate intake had a 44% lower risk of developing breast cancer than women who had the lowest folate intake. Another report in the *Journal of the American Medical Association*—showed that vitamin B6 levels were correlated with lung cancer risk—that is, people who had the lowest levels of vitamin B6 in their blood had higher risks lung cancer when compared to those who took B6 supplements and had higher levels.

Vitamin D

Vitamin D—need I say more? Okay, I will——this vitally important fat-soluble vitamin is being shown to protect men and women from a variety of cancers.

It's been over 30 years since it was suggested that low levels of vitamin D leads to higher levels of cancer. Cancer mortality rates are inversely related to sunlight exposure—in the United States, people who live in the north have higher rates of cancer than people in the south.

Since vitamin D is produced in your skin from ultraviolet radiation from the sun, the idea that supplemental vitamin D can protect you from cancer makes perfect sense. In fact, it has been suggested by multiple studies that breast cancer, ovarian cancer, prostate cancer, colon cancer, brain cancer, and pancreatic cancer are directly related to vitamin D levels—the lower the levels, the higher the risk of cancer.

For instance: A study examined the hypothetical effects of giving adults in northern climates a 1,000 IU daily dose of oral vitamin D. The authors of the study concluded that besides significantly reducing cancer rates for men and women, such a program would save the U.S. health-care system between 16 billion to 25 billion dollars. Even in a trillion-dollar health-care system, that's a whole lot of money!

Vitamin E may help prevent prostate and bladder cancer

Two studies presented at the annual meeting of the American Association for Cancer Research (AACR) showed that vitamin E could protect men from prostate cancer and bladder cancer. In the first study, researchers reported that out of 29,133 Finish men aged 50 to 69, those who had the highest blood levels of the two main forms of vitamin E (alpha and gamma tocopherol) had the lowest levels of prostate cancer. Men with the highest blood levels of alpha tocopherol were 53% less likely to develop prostate cancer, while men with high levels of gamma tocopherol lowered their risk of developing prostate cancer by 39%.

The second study, conducted by researchers at the world-renowned M.D. Anderson Cancer Center, was a case-control study on men with bladder cancer, the 4th most common cancer in men. The researchers compared 468 men with bladder cancer to 534 cancer-free patients. Men who consumed food high in alpha tocopherol reduced their risk of developing bladder cancer by 42%, while men who ate alpha-tocopherol rich foods and took a vitamin E supplement reduced their risk by 44%.

Selenium: a potent cancer fighter

As magnesium is to heart disease, selenium is to cancer. Selenium is a simple mineral that has been shown in multiple studies to help prevent many types of cancer, such as prostate cancer, colon cancer and lung cancer. One of the largest studies on selenium was done in Linxian, China. Scientists studied the effects of antioxidants—including selenium—on over 25,000 adult men and women. The results were amazing: those taking selenium with other vitamins (beta-carotene and vitamin E) had a 4% decrease in esophageal cancer deaths and a 21% decrease in stomach cancer deaths.

Does calcium cause breast cancer?

Over the years, I've had some patients say to me, "Dr. Rosick, we've heard reports on the news that calcium causes breast cancer. Is that true?"

They're referring to a study done with 7,847 pre- and post-menopausal women. Over a mean follow-up time of 17.8 years, researchers looked at the women's blood calcium levels as well as the number of women who developed breast cancer. What they found was that in pre-menopausal women, high blood levels of calcium seemed to provide protection against breast cancer. However, in post-menopausal women—and especially in those who were obese—high blood levels of calcium seemed to increase the risk of breast cancer. Confusing, isn't it?

The researchers stated that they couldn't give a good reason for these conflicting results. Since other studies have shown that post-menopausal women with high intake (greater than 1,000 milligrams per day) of calcium show lower rates of breast cancer, I recommend that all women, pre- and post-menopausal, keep taking calcium supplements if they're not getting enough calcium in their diet.

Fish oil—a truly essential supplement

You've probably guessed by now that omega-3 fatty acids from fish oil are some of my favorite supplements. In addition to protecting the heart and the brain, omega-3 fatty acids play a role in cancer prevention. Studies have shown that high blood levels of omega-3 fatty acids may protect you from breast cancer, prostate cancer, colon cancer, rectal cancer and non-melanoma skin cancers. If protecting you against heart disease, Alzheimer's and strokes isn't enough, maybe this new information will persuade you to start eating fish regularly, or at least take fish oil supplements on a daily basis.

Chlorophyllin: A little green can go a long way

Chlorophyllin, a safe, inexpensive derivative of the green plant substance chlorophyll, is another of those must-take supplements. Why? Because it helps protect you against a number of environmental toxins. Studies have shown that chlorophyllin can help protect against oral, pancreatic, colon, stomach, bladder, and breast cancer. With a resume like this, all of us who live in a polluted environment (meaning unfortunately all of us) would be wise to include this natural green nutriceutical in our daily list of supplements to take.

The key is prevention!

Like so many other politically driven wars, the war on cancer has been long on slogans and promises and woefully short on results. Sadly, the body count is high and continues to rise. But until the government and government-sanctioned private organizations wake up and see the cancer-related misery and death that too many of us have witnessed, it's up to you to protect yourself and your loved ones from cancer.

Strategies to prevent cancer

1-Behavioral Tips

- Stop smoking
- Avoid risky sex
- Avoid unnecessary X-rays and CT scans
- Don't use household or lawn and garden products that contain known carcinogens
- Avoid working the midnight shift, especially if you're a woman

2-Dietary Tips

- Eat organic foods whenever possible
- Eat a diet high in colorful vegetables and fruits (at least 5 daily servings of each)
- Eat less red meat and more soy-based products
- Drink at least two glasses of organic green tea daily

- Eat one to two cups of yogurt daily
- Limit daily alcohol consumption to two drinks

3-Supplements

- Multiple anti-oxidant formula (full spectrum of carotenoids, tocopherols and tocotrienols)
- B-complex vitamin (twice daily)
- Selenium: 100-200 mcg/day
- Vitamin D: 2,000-4,000 IU/day
- Fish oil: 2-4 g/day
- Chlorophyllin: 200-400 mg/day

The Future of Preventive Medicine

A question you might be asking is "Where does preventive medicine go from here?" In our technology-driven world, it can go wherever we want it to. Of course, it's easy to get carried away with technology without thinking about how much that technology is going to cost us, financially and otherwise.

MRI mammograms: the answer to breast cancer?

Consider MRI mammograms. It's generally believed—but by no means proven by science—that women, starting at around age 40, should get yearly mammograms (X-ray images of their breasts) to help prevent breast cancer. However, some disturbing evidence shows that yearly mammograms do not do a good job of preventing breast cancer and may in fact be contributing to breast cancer.

In the face of this evidence, I've weaned myself away from recommending—and ordering—yearly mammograms for all of my female patients 40 years and older. Instead, I recommend MRI mammograms, which use magnetic energy, rather than ionizing radiation, to look inside the breasts for early signs of cancer.

"But my doctor says I still need to get regular mammograms," you may be saying. If that's the case, have your doctor look up reports on MRI mammograms, like one the published in *The Lancet*. Researchers examined more than 7,300 women with both regular (x-ray) and MRI mammograms. They found that the MRI scans were significantly more effective in catching early breast cancer: MRI scans were 98% effective, while regular mammograms were only 52% effective.

"Does that mean I should only get MRI mammograms?" you might be asking. Unfortunately, there is no easy answer. While MRI scans more effectively detect early signs of breast cancer, they also produce more false positives. False positives can lead to a great deal of worry and perhaps even needless surgery. In addition, MRI mammograms are more expensive than X-ray mammograms, and some HMOs and insurance companies may deny payment for this potentially lifesaving tool. My final advice is that you talk to your doctor about MRI mammograms to see if this new technology is worthwhile for you.

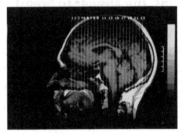

Can a brain scan detect Alzheimer's?

At the time that I finished writing this book, the only definitive way to diagnose Alzheimer's is by brain biopsy. "Now, wait a minute," you may be thinking, "A biopsy means that they take out a piece of my brain—I don't want that!"

You're right—you don't want that! Unfortunately, a brain biopsy is our best diagnostic tool for this disease. We can do non-surgical psychological tests that can give us a good idea of whether or not someone has Alzheimer's, but we can't say for sure without a biopsy. Fortunately, that may change in the near future.

Recently, scientists at the University of California, Los Angles, came up with a way to use PET (Positron Emission Tomography) scans to detect Alzheimer's as effectively as with a biopsy. A PET scan is similar to a CT scan, except that in a PET scan, a chemical is injected into your blood that allows more detailed images of your brain to be seen.

In this groundbreaking study, researchers examined 83 elderly people who had been psychologically tested for Alzheimer's. Out of the 83, 30 were thought to have Alzheimer's. Through the PET scan, the researchers showed that those 30 patients did indeed have the plaque buildup in their brains indicative of Alzheimer's.

If your memory isn't what it used to be, you might be wondering if you should go get a PET scan to check for Alzheimer's. Unfortunately, PET scans are currently very expensive, and only a few medical centers have them. However, in the future, PET scans for Alzheimer's may become as common as yearly blood tests for cholesterol.

Is genetic engineering the future of preventive medicine?

It seems that hardly a week goes by without an article or a news report about genetic engineering. While there's always undue hype about new technological wonders, genetic engineering may make prevention of chronic diseases much easier in the not-to-distant future.

The Human Genome Project (HGP), a federally and privately sponsored endeavor, has the lofty goal of deciphering our genes, which define who we are and give clues as to which chronic diseases may strike us down. In the future, your doctor may use genetic screening to spot early signs of cancer.

In fact, medical researchers can already tell women if they're at higher risk for breast cancer or ovarian cancer. Medical researchers know that mutations in two specific genes—BRCA1 and BRCA2—indicate an increased risk of developing breast cancer or ovarian cancer. How much higher that risk is depends upon certain other factors, including the following:

- A personal history of breast cancer at a young age
- A close family member (sister, mother) with breast cancer
- A family member with breast cancer in both breasts
- A family member with the BRCA1 or BRCA2 mutation
- Ashkenazi Jewish ancestors (Eastern European descent)

Now, before you run out and ask your doctor for genetic testing, remember that the vast majority of women who develop breast cancer do not have the BRCA1 or BRCA2 mutations. Genetic testing is still crude at best, so if you're interested, please talk to your doctor and a genetic counselor.

Stem cells: Hope or Hype?

It seems that every week you can read a new story about stem cells. To hear proponents tell the story, stem cells will provide us with cures from cancer to diabetes to perhaps aging itself. On the other hand, those more skeptical state that, in reality, nothing of substance has come from stem-cell research and probably nothing ever will.

Like most everything else in medicine—as in life—the answer probably lies in-between the two extremes. While it's true that stem cell research hasn't lived up to the hype of its more enthusiastic supporters, stem cells do have the potential to change the way we deal with prevention of chronic diseases. As an example, researchers at the Texas Heart Institute are attempting to use stem cells—from the patient's own body—to restore the heart to health after it's been through the ravages of heart disease and even a heart attack. Whether or not stem cell research will provide us with longer, healthier lives is unknown, but it's research that I think very well might lead to some important weapons in the fight against chronic diseases.

Epigenetics: science proves supplements are worthwhile!

If you are still not convinced, in spite of all the evidence I've presented, that proper nutritional supplements are essential in preventing the top killers of the twenty-first century, then you need to know about a new field of genetics called epigenetics. Epigenetics examines how natural biochemicals in foods such as broccoli, grapes, and lemons—foods known for their cancer-preventive properties—can stop cancer at the genetic level.

For example, researchers have shown that sulforaphanes, which are key constituents of cruciferous vegetables, may inhibit a group of enzymes that turn cancer-suppressing genes on and off. In short, the food you eat and the supplements you take may be working at the level of your DNA to prevent cancer, heart disease and other age-related aliments. While epigenetics is still in its early stages, I have no doubt that you'll be reading a lot more about this discipline in the coming years.

Supplements, supplements—where to find supplements?

One of the most frequent questions I get from patients is where to get good supplements. Unfortunately, the answer isn't as easy as directing them to the nearest health food store. You see, unlike prescription medications, there's not a single oversight group—like the FDA—that ensures the quality of vitamins and supplements. That means that you and I—the consumers of supplements—are somewhat at the mercy of the supplement manufacturers and suppliers in regards to what we're getting.

I get around this by suggesting supplements from companies and suppliers I've used for years and trust. How do I determine this? Well, for one, if they've been in the business for decades, that probably means they're putting out a reasonably good product.

You can also buy supplements online. Life Extension (www.lifeextension.com) is a well-known supplement company that I recommend and use myself. Life Extension has earned the GMP (Good Manufacturing Practices) certification from NSF International, a 3rd-party certification program of things such as cleanliness and sanitation of fulfillment facilities; in addition, Life Extension supplements are also regularly tested by independent labs for heavy metals and other contaminants. They also publish an excellent magazine detailing the latest advances in anti-aging & holistic medicine, one that I always read cover-to-cover. For just probiotics I can recommend Pure Research Products LLC (www.delimmune.com). They produce some excellent and very innovative probiotics for both intestinal health and immune functioning. When buying supplements, talk to physicians and other practitioners who have spent significant time in the holistic medicine field and who know which supplements are worthwhile and which aren't. There's no reason to waste your hard-earned money on products that won't help and may even cause you harm.

An Ounce of Prevention is Worth a Pound of Cure

When I started this book, I wanted to write something that was backed by the latest scientific studies and yet easy to read, even for those without a medical background. Hopefully, I've succeeded. I hope you've enjoyed reading this book as much as I've enjoyed writing it, and I sincerely hope that it helps put you on a path to enjoying a long, happy and healthy life.

It seems that in our modern world, people tend to discard or ignore that which isn't new and shiny. However, it would be foolish to discard the wisdom of our elders; remember, it was they who told us that "an ounce of prevention is worth a pound of cure." After researching and writing this book, I can honestly say that no truer words have ever been spoken.

Appendix

Preventive and holistic medicine organizations

Another great way to learn about preventive and holistic medicine is to investigate the many organizations devoted to this area of medicine. Below are descriptions of a few of the most well-known—and well-respected—organizations (most of which I belong to), along with their Web addresses. You can also do an Internet search for preventive and holistic medical organizations—there are many places on the Internet highway that I've never traveled to, and some may hold real gems of information.

American Botanical Council (www.herbalgram.org)

For information on herbal medicine, the American Botanical Council and its Web site can't be beat. The American Botanical Council also publishes *Herbalgram*, a magazine full of useful information on herbal medicine that I read every month.

American Holistic Medical Association
(www.holisticmedicine.org)

The American Holistic Medical Association is one of the largest and oldest organizations dedicated to bringing professionalism to the holistic medical field. While their Web site isn't comprehensive, it does provide useful information, including a list of doctors like myself who are board certified in holistic medicine.

Dr. Jonathan V. Wright's Nutrition and Healing
(www.wrightnewsletter.com)

I believe Dr. Jonathan Wright is one of the leaders and pioneers of the preventive/integrative medicine field. He puts out a wonderful newsletter that's loaded with the latest information about prevention and integrative medicine.

Cancer Prevention Coalition (www.preventcancer.com)

The Cancer Prevention Coalition is a wonderful organization founded by Dr. Samuel S. Epstein. Rather than waiting for cancer to strike you or your loved ones, head over to the Cancer Prevention Coalition's Web site and educate yourself about common-sense ways to prevent cancer. While some of the material on the site is dated, it's still worth your time.

And finally, don't forget to check out my website and blog at www.drrosick.com. I'll update it on a timely basis on all things that can affect your health and wellness, because without those two things, how can you live a truly happy life?

References

CHAPTER ONE

Grundman M, Thal L. "Treatment of Alzheimer's disease." *Neurol Clinics* 2000; 18 (4):807-28.

Mayeux R, Sang M. "Treatment of Alzheimer's disease." *New England Journal of Medicine.* 1999; 341:1670-9.

Raskind M, Peskin E. "Advances in the pathophysiology and treatment of psychiatric disorders: implications for internal medicine." *Medical Clinics of North America.* 2001;85(3):803-17.

Christen Y. "Oxidative stress and Alzheimer's disease." *American Journal of Clinical Nutrition.* 2000;71(2):621-9.

Perrig WJ, Perrig P, Stahelin HB. "The relationship between antioxidants and memory performance in the old and very old." *Journal of American Geriatric Society.* 1997;45(6):718-25.

Russo A. et al. "Red wine micronutrients as protective agents in Alzheimer's-like induced insult." *Life Sciences.* 2003; 72: 2369-79.

Savaskan E. et al. "Red wine ingredient resveratrol protects from beta-amyloid neurotoxcicity." *Gerontology.* 2003; 49: 380-83.

Jang JH, Surh YJ. "Protective effect of resveratrol on beta-amyloid-induced oxidative PC12 cell death." *Free Radical Biology & Medicine.* 2003; 34(8): 1100-10.

Zhuang H. et al. "Potential mechanism by which resveratrol, a red wine constituent, protects neurons." Annals of New York Academy of Sciences. 2003; 993: 276-86.

DeFeudis FV, Drieu K. "Gingko biloba extract (EGb 761) and CNS functions: basic studies and clinical applications." *Current Drug Targets.* 2001;1(1):25-58.

Bastianetto S. "The Gingko biloba extract (EGb761) protects hippocampal neurons against cell death induced by beta-amyloid." *European Journal of Neuroscience.* 2000;12(6):1882-90.

Yao Z. "The Ginkgo biloba extract EGb761 rescues the PC12 neuronal cells from beta-amyloid-induced cell death by inhibiting the formation of beta-amyloid-derived diffusible neurotoxic ligands." *Brain Research Bulletin.* 2001;889(1-2):181-90.

Bridi R, Crossetti FP, Steffen VM, et al. The antioxidant activity of standardized extract of Gingko biloba (EGb 761) in rats. Phytother Res 2001;15(5):449-51.

Youdim KA, Joseph JA. "A possible emerging role of phytochemicals in improving age-related neurological dysfunctions: a multiplicity of effects." *Free Radical Biology & Medicine.* 2001;30(6):583-94.

Hoerr R. "Behavioural and psychological symptoms of dementia (BPSD): Effects of Egb 761." *Behavioural Psychological Pharmacopsychiatry.* 2003; 36 (Suppl 1): S56-S61.

Moreira PI, Smith MA, Zhu X, Nunomura A, Castellani RJ, Perry G. "Oxidative stress and neurodegeneration." *Annals of the New York Academy of Science.* 2005; 1043: 545-552.

Sun X, He G, Qing H, et al. "Hypoxia facilitates Alzheimer's disease pathogenesis by up-regulating BACE1 gene expression." *PNAS.* 2006; 103(49): 18727-18732.

Shi H, Kiu KJ. Cerebral tissue oxygenation and oxidative brain injury during ischemia and reperfusion. *Frontiers in Bioscience.* 2007; 1(12): 1318-1328.

Ni JW, Matsumoto K, Li HB et al. "Neuronal damage and decrease of central acetylcholine level following permanent occlusion of bilateral common carotid arteries in rat." *Brain Research.* 1995; 673(2): 290-296.

Singh KK. "Mitochondrial dysfunction is a common phenotype in aging and cancer." *Annals of the New York Academy of Science.* 2004; 1019: 260-264.

Perrig WJ, Perrig P, Stahelin HB. "The relationship between antioxidants and memory performance in the old and very old." *Journal of the American Geriatric Society.* 1997;45(6):718-25.

Zandi, PP, Anthony JC, Khachaturian AS et al. "Reduced risk of Alzheimer disease in the users of antioxidant vitamin supplements: the Cache County Study." *Arch Neuro Psychiatry.* 2004; 61(1): 82-88.

Kapelusiak-Pielok M, Adamczewska-Goncarzewicz Z, Dorszewska J, Grochowakska A. "The protective action of alpha-tocopherol on the white matter lipids during moderate hypoxia in rats." *Folia Neurobiologica.* 2005; 43(2): 103-108.

Zamin LL, Dillenburg-Pilla P, Argenta-Comiran R et al. "Protective effect of resveratrol agaisnt oxygen-glucose dprivation in organotypic hippocampal slice cultures: involvement of the P13-K pathway." *Neurobiology of Disease.* 2006; 24(1): 170-182.

Schaefer EJ, Bongard V, Beiser AS et al. "Plasma phosphatidylcholine docosahexaenoic acid content and risk of dementia and Alzheimer's disease: the Framingham Heart Study." *Archives of Neurology.* 2006; 63(11): 1545-1550.

Lim GP, Calon F, Morihara T et al. "A diet enriched with the omega-3 fatty acid docosahexaenoic acid reduces amyloid burden in an aged Alzheimer's mouse model." *Journal of Neuroscience.* 2005; 25(12): 3032-3040.

de Wilde MC, Farkas E, Gerrits M et al. "The effect of n-3 polyunsaturated fatty acid-rich diets on cognitve and cerebrovascular parameters in chronic cerebral hypofusion." *Brain Research.* 2002; 947: 166-173.

Ramasamy R, Vannucci SJ, Yan SSD et al. "Advanced glycation end products and RAGE: a common thread in aging, diabetes, neurodegeneration, and inflammation." *Glycobiology.* 2005; 15(7): 16-28.

Opara EC. "Oxidative stress, micronutrients, diabetes mellitus and its complications." *JRSM.* 2002; 122(1): 28-34.

Houstis N, Rosen ED, Lander ES. "Reactive oxygen species have a causal role in multiple forms of insulin resistance." *Nature.* 2006; 440(7086): 944-948.

Moreira PI, Smith MA, Zhu X, Nunomura A, Castellani RJ, Perry G. "Oxidative stress and neurodegeneration." *Annals of the New York Academy of Science.* 2005; 1043: 545-552.

Ott A, Stolk RP, Van Harskamp F et al. "Diabetes Mellitus and the risk of dementia: The Rotterdam Study." *Neurology.* 1999; 53(9): 1937-1942.

Lachsinger JA, Tang MX, Shea S, Mayeus R. "Hyperinsulinemia and the risk of Alzheimer's disease." *Neurology.* 2004; 63: 1187-1192.

Fishel MA, Watson S, Montine TJ. "Hyperinsulinemia provokes synchronous increases in central inflammation and beta-amyloid in normal adults." *Archives of Neurol Psychiatry.* 2005; 62: 1539-1544.

Wu G, Fang YZ, Yang S, Lupton JR, Turner ND. "Glutathion metabolism and its implications for health." *Journal of Nutrition.* 2004; 134: 489-492.

Ames BN, Shigenaga MK, Hagen TM. "Oxidants, antioxidants, and the degerative diseases of aging." *Proceedings of the National Academy of Science.* 1993; 90: 7915-7922.

Suh JH, Wang H, Liu RM, Liu JK, Hagen TM. "Alpha lipoic acid reverses the age-related loss in GSH redox status in post-mitotic tissues: evidence for increased cysteine requirement for zGSH synthesis." *Archives of Biochemstry & Biophysics.* 2004; 423: 126-135.

Bains JS, Shaw CA. "Neurodegenerative disorders in humans: the role of glutathione inoxidative stress-mediated neuronal death." *Brain Research Reviews.* 1997; 25: 335-358.

Liu H, Wang H, Shenvi S, Hagen TM, Liu RM. "Glutathione metabolism during aging and in Alzheimer's disease." *Annals of the New York Academy of Sciences.* 2004; 1019: 346-349.

Sen CK. "Nutritional biochemistry of cellular glutathione." *Journal of Nutrition and Biochemistry.* 1997; 8: 660-672.

Droge W. "Aging-related changes in the thiol/disulfide redox state: implications for the use of thiol antioxidants." *Exper Gero* 2002; 37: 1331-1343.

Samiec PS, Botsch CD, Flagg EW, Kurtz JC, Sternberg P, Reed RL, Jones DP. "Glutathione in human plasma: decline in association with aging, age-related macular degeneration, and diabetes." *Free Radical Biology & Medicine.* 1998; 24(5): 699-704.

Jones DP, Mody VC, Carlson JL, Lynn MJ, Sternberg P. "Redox analysis of human plasma allows seperation of pro-oxidant events of aging from decline in antioxidant defenses." *Free Radical Biology & Medicine.* 2002; 33(9): 1290-1300.

Asuncion JG, Millan A, Pla R, Bruseghini L, Esteras A, Pallardo FV et al. "Mitochondrial glutathione oxidation correlates with age-associated oxidative damage to mitochondrial DNA." *FASSEB Journal.* 1996; 10: 333-338.

Julius M, Lang CA, Gleiberman L, Harburg E, DiFranceisco W, Schork A. "Glutathione and morbidity in a community-based sample of elderly." *Journal of Clinical Epidemiology.* 1994; 47(9): 1021-1026.

Lang CA, Mills BJ, Lang HL, Liu MC, Usui WM Richie J et al. "High blood glutathione levels accompany excellent physical and mental health in women ages 60 to 103 years." *Journal of Laboratory & Clinical Medicine.* 2002; 140: 413-417.

Sechi G, Deledda MG, Bua G, Satta WM, Deiana GA, Pes GM, Rosati G. "Reduced intravenous glutathione in the treatment of early Parkinson's disease." *Progress in Neuro-Psychopharmacology and Biological Psychiatry.* 1996; 20(7): 1159-1170.

Witschi A, Reddy S, Stofer B, Lauterberg BH. "The systematic availability of oral glutathione." *European Journal of Clinical Pharmacology* 1992; 43(6): 667-669.

Middleton N, Jelen P, Bell G. "Whole blood and mononuclear cell glutathione response to dietary whey protein supplementation in sedentary and trained male human subjects." *International Journal of Food Science & Nutrition.* 2004; 55(2): 131-141.

Kent KD, Harper WJ, Bomser JA. "Effect of whey protein isolate on intracellular glutathione and oxidant-induced cell death in human prostate epithelial cells." *Toxicology in Vitro.* 2003; 17: 27-33.

Marshall K. "Therapeutic applications of whey protein." *Alternative Medicine Review.* 2004; 9(2): 136-156.

Guayerbas N, Puerto M, Hernanz A, Miquel J, Fuente M. "Thiolic antixoidant supplementation of the diet reverses age-related behavioural dysfunction in prematurely ageing mice." Pharm Bio Behav 2005; 80: 45-51.

Liu J, Atamna H, Kuratsune H, Ames B. "Delaying brain mitochondrial decay and aging with mitochondrial anti-oxidants and metabolites." *Annals of the New York Academy of Science.* 2002; 959; 133-166.

Kumaran S, Savitha S, Devi MA, Panneerselvam C. "L-carnitine and alpha-lipoic acid reverse the age-related deficit in glutathione redox state in skeletal muscle and heart tissue." *Mechanisms of Ageing and Development.* 2004; 125: 507-512.

Christen Y. "Oxidative stress and Alzheimer's disease." *American Journal of Clinical Nutrition.* 2000;71(2):621-9.

Lachsinger JA, Tang MX, Shea S, Mayeus R. "Hyperinsulinemia and the risk of Alzheimer's disease." *Neurology.* 2004; 63: 1187-1192.

Liu J, Atamna H, Kuratsune H, Ames B. "Delaying brain mitochondrial decay and aging with mitochondrial anti-oxidants and metabolites." *Annals of the New York Academy of Science.* 2002; 959; 133-166.

Lim GP, Chu T, Yang F et al. "The curry spice curcumin reduces oxidative damage and amyloid pathology in an Alzheimer Transgenic mouse." *Journal of Neuroscience.* 2001; 21(21): 8370-8377.

Weinreb O, Mandel S, Amit T. et al. "Neurological mechanisms of green tea polyphenols in Alzheimer's and Parkinson's diseases." *Journal of Nutritional Biochemistry.* 2004; 15: 506-516.

Maia L, Mendonca A. "Does caffeine intake protect from Alzheimer's disease?" *European Journal Neuro.* 2002; 9: 377-382.

Rondeau V, Commeges D, Jacqmin-Gadda H, Dartigues JF. "Relationship between aluminum concentrations in drinking water and Alzheimer's Disease: an 8-year followup study." *American Journal of Epi*demiology. 2000; 152(1): 59-66.

Janson J, Laedtke T, Parisi J et al. "Increased Risk of Type-2 diabetes in Alzheimer's Disease." *Diabetes.* 2004; 53: 474-481.

Quintana B, Allam MF, Serrano Del Castillo A, Fernandez-Crehuet Navajas R. "Alzheimer's disease and coffee: a quantitative review." *Neuroscience Research.* 2007; 29(1): 91-95

Hipkiss AR. "Could carnosine or related structures suppress Alzheimer's disease?" *Journal of Alzheimer's Disease.* 2007; 11(2): 229-240.

Martin BK, Szekely C, Brandt J et al. "Cognitive function over time in the Alzheimer's disease anti-inflammatory prevention trial." *Archives of Neurol Psychiatry.* 2008; 65(7): 896-905.

Llewellyn DJ, Langa K, Lang I. "Serum 25-Hydroxyvitamin D concentration and cognitive impairment." *Journal of Geriatric Neuro* 2009 Feb 4 (e-pub.)

Pike CJ, Carroll JC, Rosario ER, Barron AM. "Protective actions of steroid hormones in Alzheimer's disease." *Fron Neuroendo* 2009; 30: 239-258.

Tong M, Neusner A, Longato L et al. "Nitrosamine exposure causes insulin resistance diseases: relevance to type-2 diabetes, non-alcholigc steatohepatitits, and Alzheimer's disease." *Journal of Alzheimer's Disease.* 2009 June 19 (e-pub).

Hsiung GY, Sadovnick AD, Feldman H. "Apolipoprotein E epsilon4 genotype as a risk factor for cognitive decline and dementia: Data from the Canadian Study of Health and Aging." *CMAJ.* 2004; 171: 863-867.

Maioli M, Coveri P, Pagni C et al. "Conversion of mild cognitive impairment to dementia in elderly subjects: a preliminary study in a memory and cognitive disorders unit." *Arch Gero Geriatrics.* 2007(1): 233-241

CHAPTER TWO

Baynes JW, Thorpe SR. Glycoxidation and lipoxidation in atherosclerosis. Free Rad & Med 2000; 28(12): 1708-1716.

Schleicher E, Weigert C, Rohrbach H, Nerlich A, Bachmeier B, Friess U. Role of glucoxidation and lipid oxidation in the development of atherosclerosis. Ann NY Acad Sci 2005; 1043: 343-354.

Asif M, Egan J, Vasan S, Jyothirmayi GN, Masurekar MR et al. An advanced glycation endproduct cross-link breaker can reverse age-related increases in myocardial stiffness. PNAS 2000; 97(6): 2809-2813.

Spiteller G. Is atherosclerosis a multifactorial disease or is it induced by a sequence of lipid peroxidation reactions? Ann NY Acad Sci 2005; 1043: 355-366.

Jandeleit-Dahm KA, Lassila M, Allen TJ. Advanced glycation end products in diabetes-associated atherosclerosis and renal disease. Ann NY Acad Sci 2005; 1043; 759-766.

Oxidants, antioxidants, and the degenerative diseases of aging. Ames BN, Shigenaga MK, Hagen TM. PNAS 1993; 90(17): 7915-7922.

Sako M et al. Cardioprotection with alcohol. Ann N.Y. Acad Sci 2002; 957: 122-35.

Hung LM et al. Cardioprotective effect of resveratrol, a natural antioxidant from grapes. Cardio Research 2000; 47: 549-55.

Daviglus ML, Stamler J, Orencia AJ, et al. Fish consumption and the 30-year risk of fatal myocardial infarction. New Engl J Med 1997;336(15):1046-53.

Marckmann P, Gronbaek M. Fish consumption and coronary heart disease mortality: a systemic review of prospective cohort studies. Eur J Clin Nutr 1999;53(8):585-90.

de Wilde MC, Farkas E, Gerrits M et al. The effect of n-3 polyunsaturated fatty acid-rich diets on cognitve and cerebrovascular parameters in chronic cerebral hypofusion. Brain Res 2002; 947: 166-173.

Daviglus ML, Stamler J, Orencia A J., et al. Fish Consumption and the 30-year risk of fatal myocardial infarction. The New England Journal of Medicine 1997; 336(15): 1046-1053.

Miller M. Current prospectives on the management of hypertriglyceridemia. American Heart Journal 2000; 140(2): 232-240.

Durrington PN, Bhatnager D, Mackness, MI, et al. Omega-3 fatty acid concentrate decreased triglycerides in coronary heart disease patients treated with simvastatin. Heart 2001; 85: 544-548.

Medizinische K, Klinikum I. N-3 fatty acids and the prevention of coronary atherosclerosis. American Journal of Clinical Nutrition 2000; 71(1): 224-227.

Bucher H, Hengstler P, Schindler C, Meir G. N-3 Polyunsaturated fatty acids in coronary heart disease: A meta-analysis of randomized controlled trials. The American Journal of Medicine 2002; 112: 298-304.

Hu F, Bronner L, Willett W. et al. Fish and omega-3 fatty acid intake and risk of coronary heart disease in women. Journal of the American Medical Association 2002; 287(14): 1815-1821.

Lorgeril M, Salen P. Fish and n-3 fatty acids for the prevention and treatment of coronary heart disease: Nutrition is not pharmacology. The American Journal of Medicine 2002; 112: 316-319.

Rosenberg I. Fish-food to calm the heart. New England Journal of Medicine 2002; 346(15): 1102-1103.

Albert C, Campos H, Stampfer M. et al. Blood levels of long-chain n-3 fatty acids and the risk of sudden death. New England Journal of Medicine 2002; 346(15): 1113-1118.

Elgharib N, Chi DS, Younis W, et al. C-reactive protein as a novel biomarker. Postgrad Med 2003;114(6):39-44.

Bazzino O, Ferreiros ER, Pizarro R, et al. C-reactive protein and the stress tests for the risk stratification of patients recovering from long-standing stable angina pectoris. Am J Cardiol 2001;87(11):1235-9.

Ridker PM, Hennekens CH, Buring JE, Rifai N. C-reactive protein and other markers of inflammation in the prediction of cardiovascular disease in women. NEJM 2000;342:836-43.

Friso S, Jacques PF, Wilson PWF, et al. Low circulating vitamin B$_6$ is associated with elevation of the inflammation marker C-reactive protein independently of plasma homocysteine levels. Circulation 2001;103:2788-91.

Ford ES, Liu S, Mannino DM, et al. C-reactive protein concentration and concentrations of blood vitamins, carotenoids, and selenium among United States adults. Eur J Clin Nutr 2003; 57 (9):1157-63.

Church TS, Earnest CP, Wood KA, Kampert JB. Reduction of C-reactive protein levels through use of a multivitamin. Am J Med 2003;115:702-7.

von Schacky C. n-3 Fatty acids and the prevention of coronary atherosclerosis. Am J Clin Nutr 2000;71(1):224-7.

Roach GW, Kanchuger M, Mangano CM., et al. Adverse cerebral outcomes after coronary bypass surgery. The New England Journal of Medicine 1996; 335(25): 1857-1864.

Lerman A, Burnett JC, Higano ST, et al. Long-term L-arginine supplementation improves small-vessel coronary endothelial function in humans. Circulation 1998; 97(21): 2123-2128.

Ceremuzynski L, Chamiec T, herbaczynska-Cedro K. Effects of supplemental oral L-arginine on exercise capacity in patients with stable angina pectoris. American Journal of Cardiology 1997; 80(3): 331-333.

Sozykin AV, Noeva EA, Balakhonova TV, et al. Effect of L-arginine on platelet function, endothelial function and exercise tolerance in patients with stable angina pectoris. Terapevticheskii Arkhiv 2000; 72(8): 24-27.

Fujita H, Yamabe H, Yokoyama M. Effect of L-arginine administration on myocardial thallium-201 perfusion during exercise in patients with angina pectoris and normal coronary angiograms. Journal of Nuclear Medicine 2000; 7(2): 97-102.

Creager MA, Gallagher SJ, Girerd XJ, et al. L-arginine improves endothelium-dependent vasodilation in hypercholseterolemic humans. Journal of Clinical Investigation 1992; 90(4): 1248-1253.

Clarkson P, Adams MR, Powe AJ, et al. Oral L-arginine improves endothelium-dependent dilation in hypercholesterolemic young adults. Journal of Clinical Investigation 1996; 97(8): 1989-1994.

Kawano H, Motoyama T, Hirai N. et al. Endothelial dysfunction in hypercholesterolemia is improved by L-arginine administration: possible role of oxidative stress. Atherosclerosis 2002; 161(2): 375-380.

Wallace AW, Ratcliffe MB, Galindez D, Kong JS. L-arginine infusion dilates coronary vasculature in patients undergoing coronary bypass surgery. Anesthesiology 1999; 90(6): 1577-1586.

Carrier M, Pellerin M, Perrault LP, et al. Cardioplegic arrest with L-arginine improves myocardial protection: results of a prospective randomized clinical trial. Annals of Thoracic Surgery 2002; 73: 837-842.

Calvert, JF. Cardiovascular disease and hypertension. Clinics in Family Practice 2001; 3(4): 733-756.

Siani A, Pagano E, Iacone R et al. Blood pressure and metabolic changes during dietary L-arginine supplementation in humans. American Journal of Hypertension 2000; 13: 547-551.

Sudden cardiac death. The American Heart Association. www.americanheart.org

Tuzcu EM, Kapadia SR, Tutar E et al. High prevalence of coronary atherosclerosis in asymptomatic teenagers and young adults. Circuation 2001; 103: 2705-2710.

Hansson GK. The stabilized plaque: will the dream come true? European Heart Jour Supplement 2001 Supplement C; 3: C69-C75.

Gensini GF, Dilaghi B. The unstable plaque. European Heart Jour Supplement 2002 Supplement B; 4: B22-B27.

Burke AP, Farb A, Malcom GT et al. Plaque rupture and sudden death related to exertion in men with coronary artery disease. JAMA 1999; 281: 921-926.

Aikawa M, Rabkin E, Sugiyama S et al. An HMG-CoA reductase inhibitor, cerivastatin, suppresses growth of macrophages expressing matrix metalloproteinases and tissue factor in vivo and in vitro. Circuation 2001; 103: 276-283.

Tompson J. Vitamins and minerals 4: overview of folate and the B vitamins. Comm Prac 2006; 79(6): 197-198.

Ye Z, Song H. Antioxidant vitamins intake and the risk of coronary heart disease: meta-analysis of cohort studies. Eur J Cardo Prev Rehap 2008; 15(1): 26-34.

48. Chen ZU, Jiao R, Ma KY. Cholesterol-lowering nutraceuticals and functional foods. Jour Ag Food Chem 2008; 56: 8671-8773.

Plat J, Mensink RP. Plant stanol and sterol esters in the control of blood cholesterol levels: mechanism and safety aspects. Am Jour Cardio 2005; 96(supp): 15D-22D.

Michos ED, Melamed ML. Vitamin D and cardiovascular disease risk. Curr Opin Nutr Metab Care 2008; 11: 7-12.

Rath M, Pauling L. Immunological evidence for the accumulation of lipoprotein(a) in the atherosclerotic lesion of the hypoascorbemic guinea pig. Proc Nat. Acad. Sci 1990; 87: 9388-9390.

Vikan T, Schirmer H, Njolstad I, Svartberg J. Endogenous sex hormones and the prospective association with cardiovascular disease and mortality in men: The Tromso Study. Eur Jour Endo 2009; 161 (3): 435-442.

Abramson, J. Overdosed America: The Broken Promise of American Medicine. Harper Perennial 2004.

CHAPTER THREE

Lee CD, Folsom AR, Blair SN. Physical activity and stroke risk: a meta-analysis. Stroke 2003; 34(10): 2475-81.

Leppala JM, Virtamo J, Fogelholm R et al. Different risk factors for different stroke subtypes: association of blood pressure, cholesterol, and antioxidants. Stroke 1999; 30: 2535-2540.

Daviglus ML, Orencia AJ, Dyer AR et al. Dietary vitamin C, beta-carotene, and 30-year risk of stroke: results from the Western Electric Study. Neuroep 1997; 16: 69-77.

Keli SO, Hertog MGL, Feskens EJM et al. Dietary flavonoids, antioxidant vitamins, and incidence of stroke: the Zutphen study. Arch Intern Med 1996; 154: 637-642.

Chang CY, Lai TJ, Lau MT et al. Plasma levels of antioxidant vitamins, selenium, and oxidative products in ischemic stroke patients as compared to matched controls in Taiwan. Free Rad Res 1998; 28: 15-24.

Juvela S, Hillborn M, Palomaki H. Risk factors for spontaneous intracerebral hemorrhage. Stroke 1995; 26: 1558-1564.

Radziszewska B, Hart RG, Wolf PA et al. Clincal research in primary stroke prevention: needs, opportunities, and challenges. Neuroepi 2005; 25: 91-104.

Krupinski J, Turu MM, Slevin M et al. Carotid plaque, stroke pathogenesis, and crp: treatment of ischemic stroke. Curr Treat Cardio Med 2007; 9(3): 229-235.

Elkind MS. Inflammation, artherosclerosis, and stroke. Neuro 2006; 12(3): 140-148.

American Heart Association. Stroke risk factors. Americanheart.org 2007.

Patrick L, Uzick M. Cardiovascular disease: C-reactive protein and the inflammatory disease paradigm. Alt Med Rev 2001; 6(3): 248-271.

Spence JD, Bang H, Chambless LE, Stampfer MJ. Vitamin intervention for stroke prevention trial: an efficacy analysis. Stroke 2005; 36: 2404-2409.

Graham IM, Daly L, Refsum H et al. Plasma homocysteine as a risk factor for vascular disease. JAMA 1997; 277: 1775-1781.

Nygard O, Nordehaug JE, Refsum H et al. Plasma homocysteine levels and mortality in patients with coronary artery disease. NEJM 1997; 337: 230-236.

Hak AE, Ma J, Powell CB et al. Prospective study of plama carotenoids and tocopherols in relation to risk ischemic stroke. Stroke 2004; 35: 1584-1588.

Wang X, Qin X, Demitras H et al. Efficacy of folic acid supplementation in stroke prevention: a meta-analysis. Lancet 2007; 369: 1876-1882.

Poole KES, Loveridge N, Barker PJ et al. Reduced vitamin D in acute stroke. Stoke 2006; 37: 243-245.

Kris-Etherton PM, Hecker KD, Bonanome A et al. Bioactive compounds in foods: Their role in the prevention of cardiovascular disease and cancer. Am J Med 2002; 113(9B): 71S-88S.

Sesso HD, Buring JE, Norkus EP, Gaziano JM. Plasma lycopene, other carotenoids, and retinol and the risk of cardiovascular disease in women. Am J Clin Nutr 2004; 79(1): 47-53.

Knekt P, Isotupa S, Rissanen H et al. Quercetin intake nad the incidence of cerebrovascular disease. Eur J Clin Nut 2000; 54(5): 415-417.

Keli SO, Hertog MG, Feskens EJ, Kromhout D. Dietary flavonoids, antioxidant vitamins, and incidence of stroke: the Zutphen study. Arch Intern Med 1996; 156(6): 637-642.

Yang CY. Calcium and magnesium in drinking water and the risk of death from cerebrovascular disease. Stroke 1998; 29: 411-414.

Mukamal KJ, Ascherio A, Mittleman MA et al. Alcohol and risk for ischemic stroke in men: the role of drinking patters and usual beverage. Ann Intern Med 2005; 142(1): 11-19.

Truelsen T, Gronbaek M, Schnohr P, Boysen G. Intake of beer, wine and spirits and risk of stroke. Stroke 1998; 29: 2467-2472.

Fraser ML, Mok GS, Lee AH. Green tea and stroke prevention: Emerging evidence. Comp Ther Med 2007; 15: 46-53.

Mozaffarian D, Longstreth WT, Lemaitre RN et al. Fish consumption and stroke risk in elderly individuals: the cardiovascular health study. Arch Intern Med 2005; 165(2): 200-206.

Rimm HE, Merchant A, Rosner BA et al. Fish consumption and risk of stroke in men. JAMA 2002; 288(24): 3130-3136.

Iso H, Rexrode KM, Stampfer MJ. Intake of fish and omega-3 fatty acids and risk of stroke in women. JAMA 2001; 285(3): 304-312.

Skerrett PJ, Hennekens CH. Consumption of fish and fish oils and dereased risk of stroke. Prev Cardio 2003; 6(1): 38-41.

Fish consumption and risk of stroke: The Zutphen study. Keli SO, Feskens EJ, Kromout D. Stroke 1994; 25(2): 328-332.

Ding EL, Mozaffarian D. Optimal dietary habits for the prevention of stroke. Sem Neuro 2006; 26: 011-023.

Fung TT, Stampfer MJ, Manson JE. Prospective study of major dietary patterns and stroke risk in women. Stroke 2004; 35: 2014-2019.

Johnsen SP, Overvad K, Stripp C et al. Intake of fruit and vegetable and the risk of ischemic stroke in a cohort of Danish men and women. Am J Clin Nutr 2003; 78: 57-64.

Moskowitz D. A comprehensive review of the safety and efficacy of bioidentical hormones for the management of menopause and related health risks. Alt Med Rev 2006; 11(3): 208-223.

Yeap BB, Hyde A, Osvaldo P et al. Lower testosterone levels predict incident stroke and transient ischemic attack in older men. J Clin Endo Metab 2009; 94(7): 2353-2359.

CHAPTER FOUR

Kelly GS. Insulin resistance: lifestyle and nutritional interventions. Alt Med Rev 2000; 5(2): 109-132.

Moran MR, Guerrero-Romero F. Oral magnesium supplementation improves insulin sensitivity and metabolic control in type 2 diabetic subjects. Diabetes Care 2003; 26: 1147-1152.

Anderson RA, Cheng N, Bryden NA et al. Elevated intakes of supplemental chromium improve glucose and insulin variables in individuals with type 2 diabetes. Diabetes 1997; 46: 1786-1791.

Jacob S, Russ P, Hermann R et al. Oral administration of RAC-alpha lipoic acid modulates insulin sensitivity in patients with type 2 diabetes mellitus: a placebo-controlled pilot trial. Free Rad Bio Med 1999; 27: 309-314.

Anderson, RA, Broadhurst CL, Polansky MM et al. Isolation and characterization of polyphenol type-A polymers from cinnamon with insulin-like biological activity. Jour Ag Food Chem 2004; 52: 65-70.

Khan A, Safdar M, Khan MMA et al. Cinnamon improves glucose and lipids of people with type 2 diabetes. Diabetes Care 2003; 26: 3215-3218.

Qin, B, Nagasaki M, Ren M et al. Cinnamon extract prevents the insulin reistance induced by a high-fructose diet. Horm Met Res 2004; 36: 119-125

Cerillo A, Guuigliano D, Quataro A et al. Vitamin E reduction of protein glycosylation in diabetes. Diabetes Care 1993; 16: 1433-1437.

Yeh GY, Eisenberg DM, Kaptchuk TJ et al. Systematic review of herbs and dietary supplements for glycemic control in diabetes. Diabetes Care 2003; 26(4): 1277-1294.

Cheng N, Zhu X, Shi H. Follow-up survey of people in China with type 2 diabetes mellitus consuming supplemental chromium. J Trace Elem Exp Med 1999; 12: 55-60.

Turpeinen AK, Kuikka JT, Vanninen E et al. Long-term effect of acetyl-l-carnitine on myocardial 1231-MIBG uptake in patients with diabetes. Clin Auton Res 2000; 10: 13-16.

DeGrandis D, Minardi C. Acetyl-l-carnitine in the treatment of diabetic neuropathy: a long-term, randomized, placebo-controlled study. Drug R.D. 2002; 3(4): 223-231.

Ametov AS, Barinov A, Dyck PJ. The sensory symptoms of diabetic polyneuropathy are improved with alpha-lipoic acid: the SYNDEY trial. Diabetes Care 2003; 26(3): 770-776.

Forsen L, Meyer HE, Midthjell K, Edna TH. Diabetes mellitus and the incidence of hip fracture: results from the Nord-Trondelag Health Study. Diabetologia 1999; 42: 920-925.

Schwartz AV, Sellmeyer DE, Ensrud KE, et al. Older women with diabetes have an increased risk of fracture: a prospective study. Jour Clin Endo Metab 2001; 86: 32-38.

Strotmeyer ES, Cauley JA, Schwartz AV, et al. Nontraumatic fracture risk with diabetes mellitus and impaired fasting glucose in older white and black adults. Arch Internal Med 2005; 165: 1612-1617.

Ametov AS, Barinov A, Dyck PJ. The sensory symptoms of diabetic polyneuropathy are improved with alpha-lipoic acid: the SYNDEY trial. Diabetes Care 2003; 26(3): 770-776.

Anderson RA. Chromium, glucose intolerance, and diabetes. JCAN, 1998; 17(6): 548-555.

Waltner-Law ME, Wang XL, Law BK, et al. Epigallocatechin gallate, a constituent of green tea, represses hepatic glucose production. Jour Bio Chem 2002; 277 (38): 34993-34940.

Vessal M, Hemmati M, Vasei M. Antidiabetic effects of quercetin in streptozocin-induced diabetic rats. Comp Biochem Physio Toxico Pharm 2003; 135C(3): 357-364.

Anjaneyulu M, Chopra K. Quercetin, an antioxidant bioflavonoid, attenuates diabetic nephropathy in rats. Clin Exp Pharm Physio 2004; 31(4): 244-248.

Huynh NT, Tayek JA. Oral arginine reduces systemic blood pressure in type 2 diabetes: Its potential role in nitric acid generation. Journal of the American College of Nutrition 2002; 5: 422-427.

Piatti P, Monti LD, Vilsecchi G et al. Long-term oral L-arginine administration improves peripheral and hepatic insulin sensitivity in type 2 diabetic patients. Diabetes Care 2001; 24: 875-880.

Devaraj S, Jialal I. Alpha tocopherol supplementation decreases serum C-reactive protein and monocyte interleukin-6 levels in normal volunteers and type 2 diabetic patients. Free Rad Biol Med 2000; 29(8): 790-792.

Moran MR, Guerrero-Romero F. Oral magnesium supplementation improves insulin sensitivity and metabolic control in type 2 diabetic subjects. Diabetes Care 2003; 26: 1147-1152.

Qin, B, Nagasaki M, Ren M et al. Cinnamon extract prevents the insulin reistance induced by a high-fructose diet. Horm Met Res 2004; 36: 119-125.

Ratner Robert E. An update on the diabetes prevention program. Endocr Pract 2006; 12(Supp 1): 20-24.

Nicolson GL. Metabolic Syndrome and Mitochondrial function: Molectular replacement and antioxidant supplements to prevent membrane peroxidation and restore mitochondrial function. Jour Cell Bio 2007; 100: 1352-1369.

Bradley R, Oberg EB, Calabrese C et al. Algorithm for complementary and alternative medicine practice and research in type-2 diabetes. Jour Alt Comp Med 2007; 1: 159-175.

Tuomilehto J, Hu G, Bidel S et al. Coffee consumption and risk of type 2 diabetes mellitus among middle-aged Finnish men and women. JAMA 2004; 291(10): 1213-1219.

McCarty MF. Nutraceutical resouces for diabetes prevention: an update. Medical Hypoth 2005; 64: 151-158.

Thornalley PJ, Babaei-Jadidi R, Ali HA et al. High prevalence of low plasma thiamine concentration in diabetes to a marker of vascular disease. Diabet 2007;

Chiu KC, Chu A, Go VL, Saad MF. Hypovitaminosis D is associated with insulin resistance and beta cell dysfunction. Am J Clin Nut 2004; 79(5): 820-825.

Mathieu c, Gysemans C, Gulietti A, Bouillon R, Vitamin D and diabetes. Diabet 2005: 48: 1247-1257.

Azadbakht L, Kimiagar M, Mehrabi Y et al. Soy inclusion in the diet improves features of the metabolic syndrome: a randomized crossover study in postmenopausal women. Am Jour Clin Nutri 2007: 85: 735-741.

Pitas AG, Harris SS, Stark PC, Dawson-Hughes B. The effects of calcium and vitamin D supplementation on blood glucose and markers of inflammation in Nondiabetic adults. Diabetic Care 2007; 30(4): 980-986.

Stiban A, Negrean M, Stratmann B et al. Benfotiamine prevents macro-andn microvascular endothelial dysfunction and oxidative stress following a meal rich in advanced glycation end products in Individuals with type 2 diabetes. Diabetes Care 2006; 29(9): 2064-2071.

Jiang R, Manson JE, Stampfer MJ et al. Nut and Peanut butter consumption and risk of type-2 diabetes in women. JAMA 2002; 28(20): 2554-2560.

Rice D, Brannigan RE, Campbell RK et al. Men's health, low testosterone, and diabetes. Diabetes Ed 2008; 34(5): 97-112.

CHAPTER FIVE

Greenwald P. Cancer chemoprevention. British Med. Journal 2002; 324: 714-718.

Messina MJ. Legumes and soybeans: overview of their nutritional profiles and health effects. Amer Jour Clin Nutri 1999; 70(suppl): 439S-450S.

Barnes, S. Effect of genistein on in vitro and in vivo models of cancer. Jour Nutri 1995; 125(suppl): 777S-783S.

Jordan VC, Morrow M. Tamoxifen, raloxifene, and the prevention of breast cancer. Endo Review 1999; 20: 253-278.

Cummings SR, Eckert S, Krueger KA, Grady D, Powles TJ, Cauley JA, et al. The effect of raloxifene on risk of breast cancer in postmenopausal women: results from the MORE randomized trial. JAMA 1999; 281: 2189-2197.

Lee HP, Gourley L, Duffy SW, Esteve J, Day NE. Dietary effects on breast cancer risk in Singapore. Lancet 1991; 337: 1197-1200.

Hirose K, Tajima K, Hamajima N. A large-scale, hospital-based case control study of risk factors of breast cancers according to menopausal status. Japan Jour Cancer Res 1995; 86: 146-154.

Yamamoto S, Sobue T, Kobayashi M, Sasaki S, Tsugane S. Soy, isoflavones, and breast cancer risk in Japan. Jour Nat Cancer Institute 2003; 95(12): 906-913.

Setchell KDR. Soy isoflavones-benefits and risks from nature's selective estrogen receptor modulators (SERMs). Jour Am College Nutri 2001; 20(5): 354S-362S.

Horn-Ross PL, John EM, Canchola AJ, Stewart SL, Lee MM. Phytoestrogen intake and endometrial cancer risk. Jour Nat Cancer Instit 2003; 95(15): 1158-1164.

Spitz M, Strom Y, Yamura Y. Epidemiologic determinants of clinically relevant prostate cancer. Int Jour Cancer 2000; 89: 259-264.

Zhou JR, Gugger ET, Tanaka T, Guo Y, Blackburn GL, Clinton SK. Soybean phytochemicals inhibit the growth of transplantable human prostate carcinoma and tumor angiogenesis in Mice. Jour Nutri 1999; 129: 1628-1635.

Jacobsen BK, Knutsen SF, Fraser GE. Does high soy milk intake reduce prostate cancer incidence? The Adventist Health Study (United States). Cancer Causes and Controls 1998; 9: 553-557.

Schoonen WM, Salinas CA, Lambertus ALM et al. Alcohol consumption and risk of prostate cancer in middle-aged men. International Jour Cancer 2004; 25: Online publication.

Wei H, Saladi R, Lu Y, Wang Y, Palep SR, Moore J, et al. Isoflavone genistein: photoprotection and clinical implications in dermatology. Jour Nutri 2003; 133(suppl): 3811S-3819S.

Cohen JH, Kristal AR, Stanford JL. Fruit and vegetable intakes and prostate cancer risk. Jour Nat Cancer Institute 2000: 92(1): 61-68.

Kolonel LN et al. Vegetables, fruits, legumes, and prostate cancer: A multiethnic case-control study. Cancer Epidemiology Biomarkers and Prevention 2000; 9: 795-804.

Freudenheim JL et al. Premenopausal breast cancer risk and intake of vegetables, fruits, and related nutrients. J National Cancer Institute 1996; 88: 340-48.

Hendler SS and Rorvik D, editors. Indole-3-Carbinol. PDR for Nutritional Supplements 2001: 218-220.

Rahman KMW, Aranha O, Sarkar FH. Indole-3-carbinol (I3C) induces apoptosis in tumorigenic but not in nontumorigenic breast epithelial cells. Nutr and Cancer 2003; 45(1): 101-12.

Nelson LR, Bulun SE. Estrogen production and action. Jour of Amer Acad Derm 2001; 45(3): 116-24.

Steiner MS, Raghow S. Antiestrogens and selective estrogen receptor modulators reduce prostate cancer risk. World Jour Urology 2003; 21(1): 31-6.

Muti P et al. Urinary estrogen metabolites and prostate cancer: a case-control study in the United States. Cancer Causes and Control 2002; 13(10): 947-55.

Nachshon-Kedmi M, Yannai S, Haj A, Fares FA. Indole-3-carbinol and 3.3'-diindolylmethane induces apoptosis in human prostate cancer cells. Food Chem Tox 2003; 41: 745-52.

Jeon KI et al. Pretreatment of indole-3-carbinol augments TRAIL-induced apoptosis in a prostate cancer cell line, LNCaP. FEBS Lettters 2003; 544: 246-51.

Heinonen OP, Albanes D, Virtamo J, et al. Prostate cancer and supplementation with alpha-tocopherol and beta-carotene: incidence and mortality in a controlled trial. J Natl Cancer Inst 1998;90(6):440-6.

Jiang Q, Christen S, Shigenaga MK, Ames BN. Gamma-tocopherol, the major form of vitamin E in the US diet, deserves more attention. Am J Clin Nutr 2001;74:714-22.

Helzlsouer KJ, Huang HY, Alberg AJ, et al. Association between alpha-tocopherol, gamma-tocopherol, selenium, and subsequent prostate cancer. J Natl Cancer Inst 2000;92(24):2018-23.

Jiang Q, Wong J, Fyrst H, et al. Gamma-tocopherol of combinations of vitamin E forms induce cell death in human prostate cancer cells by interrupting sphingolipid synthesis. PNAS 2004; 101(51): 17825-17830.

Weinstein SJ, Wright ME, Pietinen P et al. Serum alpha-tocopherol and gamma tocopherol in relation to prostate cancer risk in a prospective study. Jour Nat Cancer Inst 2005; 97(5): 396-398.

Steiner MS, Raghow S. Antiestrogens and selective estrogen receptor modulators reduce prostate cancer risk. World Jour Urology 2003; 21(1): 31-6.

Heinonen OP, Albanes D, Virtamo J, et al. Prostate cancer and supplementation with alpha-tocopherol and beta-carotene: incidence and mortality in a controlled trial. Journal of the National Cancer Institute 1998; 90(6): 440-446.

Gunawardena K, Murray DK, Meikle AW. Vitamin E and other antioxidants inhibit human prostate cancer cells through apoptosis. Prostate 2000; 44(4): 287-295.

Redman C. Inhibitory effect of selenomethionine on the growth of three selected human tumor cell lines. Cancer Letter 1998; 125(1-2): 103-110.

Helzlsouer KJ, Huang HY, Alberg AJ et al. Association between alpha tocopherol, gamma tocopherol, selenium, and subsequent prostate cancer. Journal of the National Cancer Institute 2000; 92(24): 2018-2023.

Hung LM et al. Cardioprotective effect of resveratrol, a natural antioxidant from grapes. Cardio Research 2000; 47: 549-55.

Schoonen WM, Salinas CA, Lambertus ALM et al. Alcohol consumption and risk of prostate cancer in middle-aged men. International Jour Cancer 2004; 25: Online publication.

Leibelt DA et al. Evaluation of chronic dietary exposure to indole-3-carbinol and absorption-enhanced 3.3'-diindolylmethane in Sprague-Dawley rats. Tox Sci 2003; 74: 10-21.

Athar M. Oxidative Stress and experimental carcinogenesis. Indian J Exp Bio 2002; 40(6): 656-667.

Valko M, Izakovic M, Mazur M, Rhodes CJ, Telser J. Role of oxygen radicals in DNA damage and cancer incidence. Molec and Cellular Biochem 2004; 266: 37-56.

Abe R, Shimizu T, Sugawara H, Watanabe H, Nakamura H, Choei H et al. Regulation of human melanoma growth and metastasis by AGE-AGE receptor interactions. J Inves Derm 2004; 122: 461-467.

Yamamoto Y, Yamagashi S, Hsu Cc, Yamamoto H. Advanced glycation endproducts-receptor interactions stimulate the growth of human pancreatic cancer cells through the induction of platlet-derived growth factor-B. Biochem Biophys Res Comm 1996; 222(3): 700-705.

Heijst JWJV, Niessen HWM, Hoekman K, Schalkwijk CG. Advanced glycation end products in human cancer tissues. Ann NY Acad Sci 2005; 1043: 725-733.

Galan P, Briancon S, Favier A, Bertrais S, Preziosi P et al. Antioxidant status annd risk of cancer in the SU.VI.MAX study. Bri Jour Nutr 2005; 94(1): 125-132.

Qiu JL, Chen K, Zheng JN, Wang JY, Zhang LJ, Sui LM. Nutritional factors and gastric cancer in Zhoushan Islands, China. World J Gastro 2005; 28(11): 4311-4316.

Singh KK. Mitochondrial dysfunction is a common phenotype in aging and cancer. Ann NY Acad Sci 2004; 1019: 260-264.

Miquel J. Can antioxidant diet supplementation protect against age-related mitochondrial damage? Ann NY Acad Sci 2002; 959: 508-516.

Wu G, Fang YZ, Yang S, Lupton JR, Turner ND. Glutathion metabolism and its implications for health. J. Nutr 2004; 134: 489-492.

Ames BN, Shigenaga MK, Hagen TM. Oxidants, antioxidants, and the degerative diseases of aging. Proc Nat Acad Sci 1993; 90: 7915-7922.

Suh JH, Wang H, Liu RM, Liu JK, Hagen TM. Alpha lipoic acid reverses the age-related loss in GSH redox status in post-mitotic tissues: evidence for increased cysteine requirement for zGSH synthesis. Arch Biochem Biophysics 2004; 423: 126-135.

Julius M, Lang CA, Gleiberman L, Harburg E, DiFranceisco W, Schork A. Glutathione and morbidity in a community-based sample of elderly. J Clin Epidemiol 1994; 47(9): 1021-1026.

Lang CA, Mills BJ, Lang HL, Liu MC, Usui WM Richie J et al. High blood glutathione levels accompany excellent physical and mental health in women ages 60 to 103 years. J Lab Clini Med 2002; 140: 413-417.

Witschi A, Reddy S, Stofer B, Lauterberg BH. The systematic availability of oral glutathione. Eur J Clin Pharm 1992; 43(6): 667-669.

Kent KD, Harper WJ, Bomser JA. Effect of whey protein isolate on intracellular glutathione and oxidant-induced cell death in human prostate epithelial cells. Toxi Vitro 2003; 17: 27-33.

Marshall K. Therapeutic applications of whey protein. Alt Med Review 2004; 9(2): 136-156.

Bounous G. Whey protein concentrate and glutathione modulation in cancer treatment. Anticancer Res 2000; 20(6C): 4785-4792.

Maillard V, Bougnoux P, Ferrari P, et al. n-3 and n-6 Fatty acids in breast cancer adipose tissue and relative risk of breast cancer in a case-control study in Tours, France. Int J Cancer 2002;98:78-83.

Wolk A, Larsson SC, Johansson JE, Ekman P. Long-term fatty fish consumption and renal cell carcinoma incidence in women. JAMA 2006; 296(11): 1371-1376.

Provost D, Cantagrel A, Lebailly P et al. Brain tumours and exposure to pesticides: a case-control study. Occ Prev Med 2007; 64(8): 509-514.

Surh YJ. Anti-tumour promoting potential of selected spice ingredients with antioxidative and anti-inflammatory activities: a short review. Food Chem Tox 2002; 1091-1097.

Kuhl CK, Schrading S, Bieling HB et al. MRI for diagnosis of pure ductal carcinoma in situ: a prospective observational study. Lancet 2007; 370(9586): 485-492.

Naganuma T, Kuriyama S, Kakizaki M et al. Green tea consumption and hematological malignancies in Japan. The Ohsaki Study. Amer Jour Epidem 2009 170(6): 730-738.